THE
MIRACLE
OF
WINE

By the same author:

DINE OUT AND LOSE WEIGHT

EAT YOURSELF SLIM

THE MONTIGNAC METHOD – Just for Women

RECIPES AND MENUS

MONTIGNAC PROVENÇALE COOKBOOK

EAT WELL AND STAY YOUNG

The books of Michel Montignac are also available in the following languages:

DUTCH, FINNISH, FRENCH, GERMAN, ITALIAN, RUSSIAN and SPANISH.

For further information regarding the Montignac dietary method, please contact:

Montignac Publishing UK Ltd.

Tel: +44 (0)1277 218616
Fax: +44 (0)1277 216591

The Montignac Food Range and other foods compatible with the Montignac Method, including books, are obtainable from:

Montignac Food Boutique & Café
160 Old Brompton Road LONDON SW5 0BA

Tel/Fax: +44 (0)171 370 2010
E-mail: ehilton@netcomuk.co.uk

MICHEL MONTIGNAC

THE
MIRACLE
OF
WINE

Translated from the original French version
Boire du vin pour rester en bonne santé

MONTIGNAC PUBLISHING UK

The publisher would like to thank
Wendy Jarrett
Jasminka Jenkins
Graham Webb
for their invaluable help in preparing
this book for publication.

"The Miracle of Wine"
First Published 1998
by
Montignac Publishing UK Ltd
1 Lumley Street
LONDON W1Y 2NB

First published in France under the title:
Boire du vin pour rester en bonne santé
1997

Text © Nutrimont/Montignac Publishing UK Ltd.
Front cover illustration ©: CHRISTIE'S IMAGES. Artist: Michelangelo Merisi da Caravaggio.
Interior colour illustrations ©:
Colour section 1: pgs 1-3, CEPHAS/Mick Rock; pg 4, CEPHAS/WINE Magazine
Colour section 2: CEPHAS/Mick Rock
Colour section 3: pgs 1/4, CEPHAS/Mick Rock; pgs 2-3, CEPHAS/Nigel Blythe
Colour section 4: pg 1, CEPHAS/Stockfood 090SS02223;
pgs 2-3, CHRISTIE'S IMAGES. Artist: Peder Severin Kroyer;
pg 4, CHRISTIE'S IMAGES. Artist: Preyer Johann Wilhelm.

Translated by Stuart Rothey.

ISBN 2 90 6236 64 0

Interior by Design/Section, Frome.
Printed and bound by Butler & Tanner Limited,
Frome and London.

List of Contents

List of Tables

LIST OF CHARTS

INTRODUCTION

Sunday 17 November, 1991. It is almost seven o'clock in the evening and 40 million faithful viewers are settling down to see their favourite CBS programme "Sixty Minutes".

An hour later, America is in a state of shock. It has just heard the results of a huge and lengthy comparative study conducted by the World Health Organisation, regarding the different risk factors affecting heart disease in every country in the world.

In this study, one country – France – stands out from the rest as it has the lowest incidence of cardio-vascular disease of them all. Out of the blue, the "French Paradox" is born!

This news is particularly perplexing for the Americans. Until now, they have always been told that cardiovascular disease is closely linked to high levels of cholesterol in the blood brought about by eating too much fat. And now they are told that the French, who eat as much fat as the Americans and have an average cholesterol level which is almost identical, have an incidence of cardiovascular disease that is three times lower than that recorded in the United States.

"How can this be?" the viewers ask themselves. And the scientists' answer comes like a bombshell. "It is because the French drink wine – eleven times as much as the Americans!"

"Quite clearly" the scientists say, "wine protects against cardiovascular disease, which is one of the principal causes of death in the Western world today."

This is a revelation to the public. However, it comes as no great surprise to the scientists who have been working on the subject for many years.

Even as early as 1786, the English doctor Herbeden had noted that wine relieved the pain associated with pectoral angina. And although in the more recent past, talking about the beneficial effects of wine on health would have been considered a joke in the worst possible taste, there has been ample scientific and medical documentation to show that wine is beneficial for the cardio-vascular system.

At first, it seemed that the alcoholic content of wine was the element responsible. As a result, there were those who maintained that all

13

alcoholic drinks had the same effect as wine. However, many studies have shown that this is not the case. Only wine has a positive effect on cardio-vascular disease, though it must be stressed that its beneficial qualities can only have full effect when it is drunk on a regular basis (at each principal meal) and in moderate quantities (two to four glasses a day).

Heavy drinking on an irregular basis, say at weekends, has no beneficial effect at all. On the contrary, it can be dangerous because the lack of alcohol in the bloodstream on Monday can result in a thickening of the blood, leading to clots and possibly heart attacks.

The health-giving properties of wine have been widely known since ancient times but seem to have been passed over with the coming of modern medicines.

However, current scientific studies are helping us to rediscover the healing qualities of wine – how it acts as a powerful brake on the ageing process, helps combat stress, improves digestion and fights infection.

So the French should be proud that their country is seen today by the rest of the world as a model of healthy living and they should be proud of its contribution to perpetuating and improving the art of wine making over the last 2,000 years. Not only has France helped preserve an important part of man's heritage, it has also created for itself one of the finest jewels in its economy and its culture.

Unfortunately, however, France and its paradox are drifting apart.

For just as those who have introduced us to the charms of fizzy drinks and cola are telling us why the French are in better health than they are themselves, France is in the process of renouncing its culture and throwing its wine making tradition onto the scrap heap.

As a result of campaigns against alcohol, in which the ill-informed use wine as a focus for their anger, the fruit of the vine is rapidly losing the noble image and associations it has enjoyed for centuries. In passing laws which echo the worst aspects of prohibition, France stands accused of burning its saints at the stake of political correctness. And further, by making moderate but regular wine drinkers feel guilty about their habit, the public authorities not only injure the wine industry, they also undermine the long-term health of their citizens.

Under the pretext of reducing alcohol dependency, the many campaigns that have been undertaken by the French government over the last 40 years have had the effect of halving the national consumption of wine whilst leaving the number of alcoholics as high as it was at the start.

And what is particularly interesting is that there is virtually no alcoholism associated with wine in France. In fact, in the wine-producing areas of Bordeaux and Burgundy, the incidence of alcoholism is at its lowest, whereas in the regions of Brittany and Calais, where there is not a vine to be seen, alcoholism is at its highest.

It is time for the French to take stock, for if the public authorities do not take effective measures to inform and educate the nation – particularly the young – this national heritage will be relegated to regional museums, to survive only in books and glossy magazines. And the young will die of heart attacks at the same rate as the Americans do today.

Let us hope, therefore, that this book will help both the French and the rest of the world become much more aware of this precious gift they have inherited – the miracle which is called wine.

It is a legacy we have a duty to preserve and pass on to future generations, not only for their pleasure but also for their lasting health.

CHAPTER 1

WINE – SYMBOL OF CIVILISATION

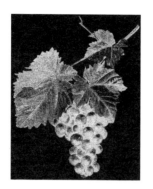

"The history of wine cannot be separated from the history of humanity. Wine, fruit of the vine and the labour of man, is no mere drink. Companion to man over the ages, wine contains something of the sacred and something of the profane.

It is a testament to civilisation and is a measure of the quality of life. It is a cultural asset. It is a factor of social life."

Anyone would think that this lyrical flight of fancy is the impassioned declaration of a wine buff sounding off about his favourite tipple.

Not at all!

This text, which could well have been taken from the speech of a grand master of a wine fraternity at his installation, is nothing more than a passage drawn from an official communiqué issued by the French delegation to a meeting at a European Commission in Brussels in 1990.

It quite clearly says that wine is different from other drinks. Considered for a long time to be almost a food, it is surrounded by a rich symbolism comparable to that of bread, with which it is often associated.

Wine is a universal symbol, with its own language linking man, the world and the mystery of life. What is more, its history is intimately connected with man, whose existence in Genesis is associated with the vine, the tree of life.

From the immortal brew in Greek mythology, to the joy and friendship of contemporary rites by way of Christ's blood in the Christian liturgy, the symbol of wine has made its presence felt for thousands of years because its roots are sacred.

And yet this drink of the gods, and subsequently of God himself, has become that of men. For the first time in its eternal history, it is now put to a severe test by a group of fanatics who can only see in its alcoholic vapours the seal of Satan.

THE WINE OF MYTHOLOGY

The origins of wine are to be found in Transcaucasia, developing later in India. From the regions in India, wine (from the Sanskrit word meaning

19

"loved") extends around the Mediterranean basin, where it was to become the object of a divine trilogy: Osiris-Dionysos-Bacchus.

In Egypt it is the Râ, the sun god and creator of the world, who introduces wine on earth. He makes this drink to preserve the human race from the anger of Hathor. Later, Egyptian mythology brings together Râ, the day sun, and Osiris, the night sun. Wine is then consecrated to Osiris from the day of his birth, when the waters of the Nile were transformed into wine. When Osiris was killed, his body was cut up into 26 pieces and thrown into the river. The revitalising effect of nectar was so strong that Osiris was brought back to life after Isis sewed his body together again.

In Greece all the symbolism of wine was expressed through Dionysos, the son of Zeus. Long before Jesus Christ, wine is linked to the blood of the god who, on 6 January each year, changes water into wine in the temple on the island of Andros.

Dionysos was particularly glorified once a year during the spring festivities. On the first day, the wines of all the landowners were consecrated to the gods in the sanctuary, after which the amphorae were opened so that the new wine could be tasted. The second day was consecrated to competitions and the man who managed to drink a pitcher of wine faster than anyone else was declared the winner. There then followed a sort of carnival, in which a giant phallus was paraded, and the *basilinna*, queen of the festival, was united in the flesh with a man representing Dionysos. This royal coupling was a fertility rite and a renewal of spring. The funerary libations followed on the third day in honour of the departed and to ensure their benevolence towards the crops and particularly the vine.

Thus it was that the Dionysan festivities were conducted under the sign of rebirth through wine, the brew of immortality, but also under the sign of sexual potency and the fecundity of nature. For the cult of Dionysos always had this double dynamic: an ascent towards the sky for fusion with the divine on the one hand and a descent towards earth, the nourishing mother, on the other.

But if Dionysos symbolised order for the Greeks, Bacchus for the Romans, in the famous Bacchanalia, is more evocative of drunkenness, luxury and social disorder.

This festival, dedicated to the god of wine, went on for several days – taboos disappeared and virtually everything was allowed. It was possible to say anything and do almost anything. The divisions between social classes disappeared and real social integration was achieved. In the centuries that followed, this ancient festival continued to survive in the guise of the carnival.

In this way the Romans institutionalised an annual ritual transgression to enable them to accept order for the rest of the time. Freud summed it up when he said:"The Festival is an organised disorder which re-enforces order."

Today it really seems that we have lost this joyous feeling for the festival. The cult of the individual, the by-product of urbanisation, has certainly contributed to this loss.

Modern society glorifies above all what is rational because it now only believes in science. Symbolism, which once gave meaning and illuminated man's life, has now evaporated in the cold light of reason, just as the morning mists evaporate in the cold light of dawn. Reason has made man into an orphan, cutting him off in turn from the earth, nature and the universe – to which he now relates in material rather than in spiritual terms.

If new generations do not drink wine but rather prefer fizzy drinks and sugary colas, it is in part because they are the victims of a continuing process of demystification, brought about by an industrial society hell-bent on development at all costs.

And yet wine, a fundamental part of our civilisation, still manages to survive in a modern world, though unfortunately it does not seem to have captured the imagination of the young. These live in urban areas that bear little relationship to the ideal city, of which Plato said:"The citizens will produce grain and wine, clothes and shoes, and will build houses. They and their children will rejoice in drinking wine, carrying garlands and singing praises to the gods."

It is predicted that the twenty-first century will be more spiritual than this one. However, this is by no means certain – unless, of course, the gods who are currently fashionable disappear into oblivion.

WINE IN THE JUDEO-CHRISTIAN WORLD

Discussion persists about the nature of the sacred fruit in the terrestrial paradise of the Garden of Eden. Some maintain that the famous apple was but a grape, since only the juice of the grape was capable of transforming the spirit of man. For did not the serpent say to Eve (Genesis 3:4, 5): "No, you will not die! God knows in fact that the day you eat it, your eyes will be opened and you will be like gods, knowing good from evil."

But "officially" (Genesis 9:20), it was after the purifying deluge that Noah planted the vine for the first time, as he did for the two other sacred plants of the Bible, the olive tree and the fig tree.

Thus it was that the vine, a gift from God to man, became the image of Israel. This explains how the chosen race came to be symbolised by a vine stock uprooted by God in Egypt.

To Israel who deceived him, God said one day (Isaiah 5:1–7): "O my beloved vine, I have cared for you, tilled the earth for you, pruned you and surrounded you with walls. I have hewn out of your middle a press. What more could I do for you that I have not already done? And you gave me thistles and weeds in return. Tell me, what have I done to you?"

Later, the punishment of an unfaithful Israel by God is represented by the symbolic destruction of the vine. Divine forgiveness is expressed in the same terms (Zechariah 8:12): "Now they will sow in peace; the vine will give its fruit."

The symbol of wine as the blood of life is already present in the Old Testament. The Book of Genesis (49:11) talks of the one who:"washes his clothes in wine, his robes in the blood of the grape" and the author of Deuteronomy (32:14) talks of wine as:"the blood of the grape."

On a more profane note, the book of Ecclesiasticus (31:27) claims that: "Wine gives life when drunk in moderation."

What a life then for a man without wine! Wine has been created to make men happy, to warm their hearts and illuminate their souls.

In the Song of Songs (7:9–11), wine is the sign of the union between man and woman: "May your breasts be clusters of grapes, your breath sweet-scented as apples, and your palate like sweet wine. Flowing down the throat of my love, as it runs on the lips of those who sleep. I belong to my love and his desire is for me."

Thus we find in the Bible a double language regarding wine: the apology for a sacred drink, the source of harmony and symbol of the relation between man and God, but also a very clear warning against the risks of abuse.

Among the seven deadly sins, it is drunkenness to which God makes specific reference when denouncing the sin of gluttony.

In the New Testament, it is certainly not by chance that Jesus accomplished his first miracle in transforming water into wine during the marriage at Cana.

Moreover, the vine was a permanent point of reference for Jesus. When explaining for example, how man relates to God, John (15:1,5) recalls his words: "I am the true vine and my Father is the vinedresser I am the vine, you are the branches."

It is during the Last Supper, the famous sign of communion between Jesus and his disciples, that the significance of wine is made apparent. Jesus laid down the foundations of Christianity when he took the cup of wine and said (1 Corinthians 11:25): "This cup is the new covenant in my blood. Whenever you drink it, do this as a memorial of me."

It was in this way that the transformation of wine into the blood of Christ and bread into his body gave birth to the Eucharist, the first sacrament of the Christian religion. And it was because Jesus said (John 6:56): "Whoever eats my flesh and drinks my blood, lives in me and I live in that person" that the elements of communion continued to be given in both forms in the mass until the fifteenth century.

But Jesus also added during the Last Supper (Matthew 26:28): "For this is my blood, the blood of the covenant, poured out for many for the forgiveness of sins."

It is in this way that the blood of the cross seals the new commitment between God and men. It is precisely this blood of Christ, issuing from his pierced side on the cross and collected in a cup, which maintained the mystical quest of King Arthur and the Knights of the Round Table for the Grail that promised immortality.

What is more, when Jesus Christ declared (Mark 14:25):"I shall never drink wine any more until the day when I drink the new wine in the kingdom of God", he was anticipating that his death would be the declaration of a new era, a renaissance, a new birth.

It is thus that one comes to understand what everybody seems to have forgotten, namely how wine in the Christian tradition is not only a source of joy, peace and life, but also the link between man and God. It is an understanding not too far removed from that underlying the cult of Dionysos.

Making wine sacred as the blood of Christ together with the intuitive perception of the New Covenant, marks the beginning of a new era, while the annual festivities in honour of the Greek god mark only the rebirth of Nature with the coming of Spring.

In this latter case, the myth is by nature cyclical, whereas in the Christian tradition it is by nature cosmic, constituting a point of departure with a trajectory that leads to the inauguration of a new era.

WINE AND ISLAM

Some might believe that the ban on drinking wine is inherent to the Islamic faith. This is not the case because the Koran has never prohibited the use of wine, although it does allude to the dangers of excess in the consumption of wine and the drunkenness which follows. But in another sura, or chapter, it says: "Satan longs to incite hatred and enmity among you [men] through wine and gambling. He wants to distance you from God and prayer." It would seem therefore that it is more the fear of drunkenness which is at the origin of Muslim abstinence rather than a Koranic ban.

It is for this reason that the orthodox Sunni fundamentalists have prohibited the consumption of wine.

The schismatic Shiites have on the other hand, made it a point of honour to adopt a contrary attitude by authorising the consumption of wine, providing drunkenness is avoided. To drink wine is moreover for them sign of resistance to dogmatic fundamentalism and a way of affirming a "counter-theology".

In the eleventh century, the cultivation of the vine was particularly flourishing in Muslim countries. The famous Persian doctor Avincenna said: "Wine is the friend of the wise man and the enemy of the drunkard. It is bitter and useful; like the counsel of the philosopher, it is allowed to those with spirit but prohibited to idiots. It pushes the sot towards the shadows and guides the wise man towards God. Also, religion allows it to the wise man and reason prohibits it to the poor of spirit."

It would seem that this reasonable attitude was made more extreme by educated people for whom wine not only favoured inspiration but even lead to Revelation. Wine thus became a symbol of esoteric knowledge for the literate and was reserved for the élite and above all the initiates.

This is why people continued to drink into the twelfth century and why magnificent poems were published, such as *In Praise of Wine* by Omar Ibn Al Faridh. To these may be added the works of Omar Khayyam, who sang of wine before going back to Allah to find out how to use it, proclaiming: "To drink wine and embrace beauty, is more worthy than the hypocrisy of the devout; if the lover and the drinker of wine are doomed to hell, then no one will see the face of the sky."

The fear of death and the uncertainty of what lies beyond, prompted Omar Khayyam to Epicureanism: "Since nothing here can guarantee a tomorrow, make your lovesick heart happy now in the light of the moon, by drinking wine; for this star will search for us tomorrow and will see us no more."

The theme of rebirth through wine is also to be found in Omar Khayyam's writing, but in an original form when he says: "After my death, make sure you have a cup or jar with my dust; fill it with wine and perhaps I will live again."

However, if wine guides the initiate, it also, according to Khayyam, allows the profane access a higher knowledge; he affirms: "I know that only wine has the word of the enigma and that it brings awareness of a perfect unity." Wine thus allows access to a hidden truth.

As far as the poet and philosopher Hafiz was concerned, he believed that drinking wine integrated man in the movement of the universe and thus made him belong to the cosmos.

25

CHAPTER 2

THE USE OF WINE OVER THE AGES

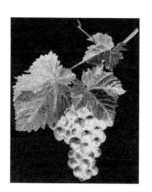

Like all myths, the origins of wine are lost in the mists of time.

However, by studying ancient texts and particularly through archaeology, we have come to know quite a lot more about how wine was produced, how it was drunk in various civilisations and where and how it developed.

WINE IN THE ANCIENT WORLD

Wine in Egypt

Egypt was the first country to develop the vine in the area surrounding the Mediterranean. Numerous bas-reliefs that survive from ancient times bear testimony to this fact. However, it would appear that it was not in widespread use because, owing to its sacred nature, wine was used mainly in religious ceremonies – for example, funerary wine. In fact it was drunk only by religious dignitaries or politicians. The pharaoh drank it, but apparently he preferred beer, like his subjects.

Wine in Greece

Wine was widely drunk in Ancient Greece, where the meals were organised rather differently from our own.

Breakfast consisted of barley bread soaked in undiluted wine, followed at lunchtime, by a snack of bread, olives and some fruit. Supper occurred fairly early in the afternoon, was much more important and evolved in three phases. Firstly, there was an aperitif consisting of aromatic wine served in a large cup, which was then passed round the group from one person to the other. The meal started after this, beginning with meats and cereals. Only water was drunk at this stage. The third and most important part followed, when little was eaten apart from some bread rolls and dried fruit, but plenty of wine was drunk.

Only the men stayed on for this part of the meal, which was called the *symposium*. The few women present were either dancers or courtesans and wine was drunk during the course of this adjunct to the meal, following a well-defined ritual.

29

The participants started with a libation to Dionysos to whom, as mentioned above, men were indebted for the gift of wine. First of all, each person drank a mouthful of undiluted wine, then a few drops were poured onto the ground invoking the name of the deity. Following this, the "king of the banquet" was chosen by casting lots: it was his task to decide on the ratio of water that should be poured into the special vessels of wine called "craters". In Ancient Greece, wine was rarely drunk without water because it was so thick.

Then the *symposium* began (literally "the act of drinking together"), when those assembled would start to discuss and philosophise on a topic chosen by the king of the banquet. During these cogitations, everyone would listen to the music, watch the dancers, hear the poets recite their works and generally exercise their minds whilst continuing to drink wine. Wine was drunk and bread was broken and eaten in a climate of "peace and affection", as is still done today at meetings of brotherhoods and masons. These *agape* meals fostered feelings of solidarity and brotherhood between men and could last for hours, but they would always conclude before nightfall, at the setting of the sun.

The Ancient Greeks produced various different wines – aromatic wines, wines mixed with honey, thyme, mint or cinnamon. They even cooked wines. Gradually they started to produce fine wines. Odysseus, for example, mocked the second-rate wine offered by the Cyclops Polyphemus which he judged unworthy of the Greek world. Wine transported by sea was stored in amphorae; by land, the heavy earthenware containers were replaced by goatskins sealed with pitch. Some wines lasted several years: in the *Odyssey,* King Nestor drank a wine that was eleven years old.

Wine in Rome

According to Roman tradition, wine was introduced by Saturn, the god of sowing and of the vine, whose symbols were the sickle and the pruning knife. Only later was wine associated with Bacchus.

The Ancient Romans were actively involved in perfecting the techniques of wine making. As a result, they managed to create wines that could be aged for 20 years or more. The wine was poured into amphorae of 26 litres which were labelled with the area of production and the year it was stored. Horace even speaks of a wine that was 60 years old and Pliny the Elder claimed to have drunk on one occasion a wine that had been stored for a couple of centuries.

Apicius, Horace, Pliny and Martial, describe in their works the many vintages that charmed ancient palates. The most important and prestigious were the wines from the Latium, Gauranum or Campania, and the most ordinary were those from Spoleto, Umbria and Plignum. Those from Salina, Ravenna or the Vatican were considered undrinkable.

However, as with the Greeks, the Romans considered wine a class drink. Slaves and soldiers in the lower ranks were only allowed to drink a mixture of cheap wine, vinegar and water. This is the reason Jesus on the cross had to be content with satisfying his thirst by sucking a sponge soaked in vinegar. To our eyes, this act seems somewhat bizarre, but in fact the centurion was merely offering Christ the customary tipple of the Roman soldier. On the other hand, the Romans drank many aromatic wines, which were used a great deal in cooking, as can be seen in the many recipes of the famous cook Apicius.

In the manner in which they drank wine and took their meals, the Romans owed much to Greek tradition. Wine, which was always thick, was invariably cut with water; according to Virgil, drinking wine in its natural state was what "barbarians unworthy of Bacchus" did.

Shortly after the foundation of Rome, only men over 30 years of age had the right to drink wine. Women were forbidden to drink it for a long time. Cato even said: "If you catch your wife drinking wine, kill her!". Moreover, it was the custom for the *pater familias*, the head of the household, to kiss all the women of his household on the lips each day to make certain that none of them had drunk any wine.

The Romans used to take four meals a day: the *jentaculum*, the *prandium*, the *cena* and the *vesperna*. About 200 BC, the *vesperna* disappeared fairly rapidly, leaving the *jentaculum* (a breakfast of bread, cheese and water), the *prandium* (a mid-morning snack of bread, olives and fruit) and the *cena* (see below) that became the only important meal. However, under the influence of the "hygienists", as the centuries went by Romans began to neglect the morning meals to concentrate almost exclusively on the important main meal, the *cena*. This meal took place about two o'clock in the afternoon and brought to an end the day's work that had begun at about five or six o'clock in the morning.

As with the Greeks, the Romans drank water with lavish dishes served in the *triclinium*, a sort of dining room. The group would then move to another room or rearrange the furniture, in order to organise the *commisatio* (identical to the platonic banquet) at which the men assembled to drink wine. The president of the gathering decided or determined by casting dice, not only how much water should be used to cut the wine (from a third to four-fifths at most) but also the number of cups that should be drunk by each participant. The wine was then taken from the amphora and mixed with the water in bronze or silver vessels.

Detailed studies have allowed us to discover that the Romans drank about two litres of undiluted wine per day – which would seem to be quite different from the impressions given by writings like the *Satyricon* of Petronius, in which the Bacchic orgies are so vividly described.

WINE IN FRANCE

Wine in Gaul

About 600 BC, the Phoenicians planted the first vines in Gaul in the region between Marseilles, d'Agde and Nice. However, these vines were more suited to the production of grapes than of wine.

The Gauls preferred beer made from barley or fermented milks. Until the fourth century BC, wine was reserved for warriors, but by the end of the second century BC, it was drunk more widely. It was no longer drunk solely by the élite but also by the middle classes – by traders, artisans and landowners – who brought it in from Italy. With the Roman colonisation shortly before 100 BC, many vineyards were planted in the area around Narbonne (Languedoc). However, only Roman citizens and colons (army veterans) had the right to cultivate the vine.

The Gauls rapidly acquired a taste for wine, to such an extent that a contemporary of Julius Caesar, Diodorus of Sicily, said: "they are capable of trading a slave for an amphora of wine". In fact, during the 50 years

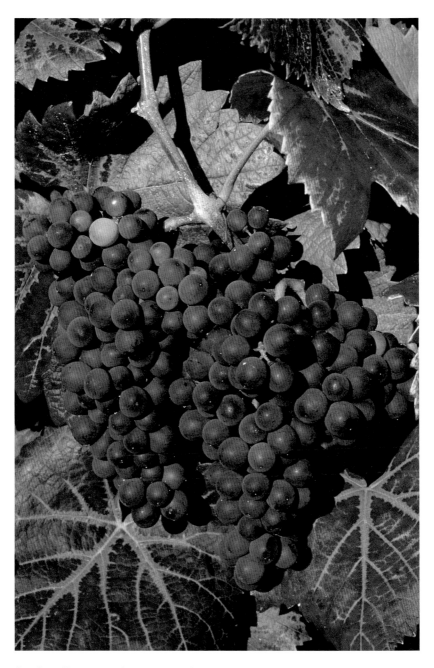

Ripe Pinot Noir grapes – here growing at Verzenay, on the Montagne de Reims, France.

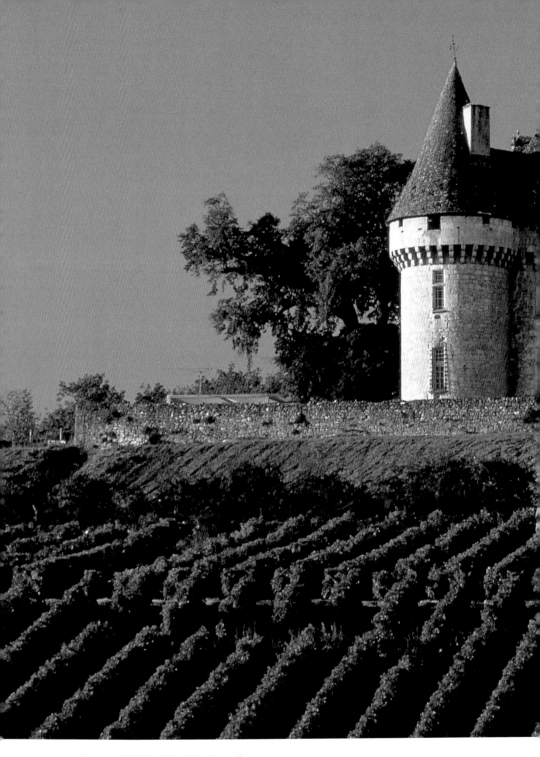

Chateau de Monbazillac, Dordogne, France.

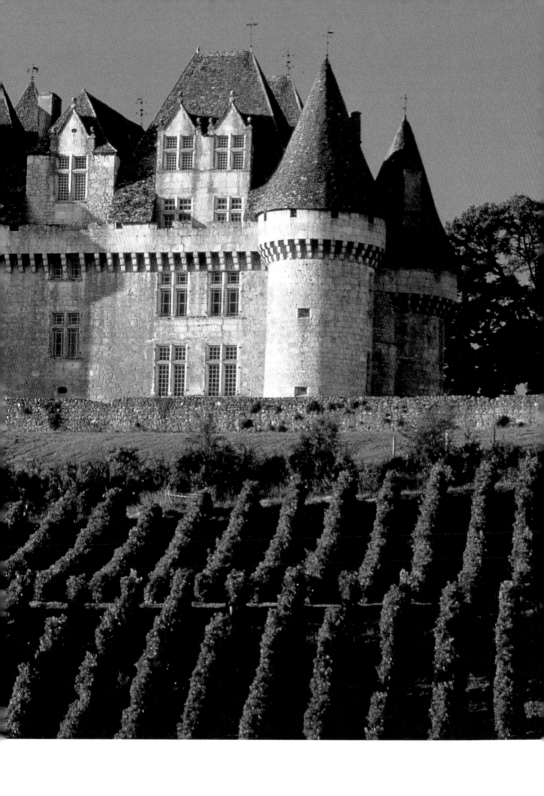

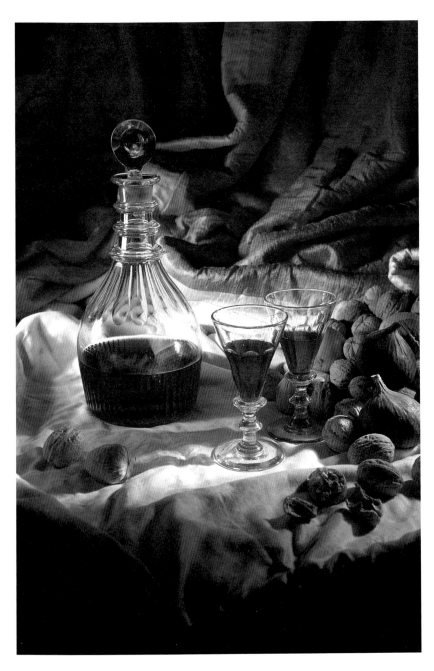

Decanter and glasses of port with figs.

between 110 BC to 60 BC, one and a half million litres of wine were imported into Gaul every year.

The Romans drank sticky wines that were resinated, smoked or flavoured with aniseed, cumin or thyme. But to their complete amazement, as they considered the practice both barbarous and scandalous, the Gauls drank unadulterated wine during the course of a meal, from the horn of an aurochs (a wild ox now extinct). The inscriptions found on these drinking vessels bear testimony to the symbolism associated with the use of wine during this period: "Live happy!", "May it bring you luck!", "Use it well!" or again "The more unhappy you are, the more you will drink, and the happier you are, the more you will drink!".

The wine trade was very fruitful for Rome. However, it was disrupted by the Helvetii on the Rhône-Saône route, by the Venetii in Armorica and by the Germans on the Rhine. This restriction to the trade in Roman wine was undoubtedly one of the reasons that prompted Caesar to invade Gaul in 58 BC: for him, this was the best way of ensuring that his production of wine would continue to flourish.

With the Roman conquest, the vine penetrated further and further into Gaul. It grew abundantly in Provence, in the Languedoc, in the Rhône Valley, on the Côte-d'Or and in Aquitaine. Later it appeared in Burgundy, in Lutetium (Paris) and Colonia Treverorum (Trier) on the Moselle. It took much longer to reach in the Champagne area, in the valley of the Loire and among the Jura Mountains.

The Gauls rapidly surpassed their Roman masters in the art of viticulture. Cicero tells us that the Roman Senate was sufficiently worried to proclaim that no further vines could be planted in Transalpine Gaul. This was done to preserve the trade with Gaul of Roman wine. However, it did not succeed because the proclamation was very badly implemented. In addition to improving the methods for producing wine, the Gauls developed a far superior method for conserving it when they invented the barrel in 62 BC. Shortly before the birth of Christ, the wines from Gaul were so much better than the competition that they had already begun to invade Italy.

In Gaul, the majority of people drank wine, but there was considerable variety in the quality. Only rich Gauls had access to the old, strong wines, which were drunk after they had been filtered for impurities and sediment. The functionaries, employees and soldiers drank more ordinary wines, which they bought in the taverns to drink on the premises or take back to their lodgings in terracotta flasks. The rest of the population – artisans, agricultural workers, slaves or freedmen – only had access to "Lora", a cheap wine made by treading the grape marc and allowing it to stand in its juices, or cheap wine coming from amphorae that had been badly sealed. Alternatively, they had to content themselves with water added to vinegar.

The wines from Gaul were so successful that the trade in Roman wines became critical. So in AD 92, emperor Domitian gave orders that half the vineyards in Gaul should be destroyed. This measure was probably all the more necessary because the cultivation of vines had become so widespread in Gaul that there was now a lack of wheat. However, the edict was never properly implemented and it was finally abolished in AD 280 by the emperor Probus.

In AD 392, under Theodore the Great, Christianity was declared the sole religion of the Roman Empire. Since wine was necessary for celebrating the Eucharist, this edict merely reinforced the cultivation of the vine until development was arrested in Gaul with the collapse of the Roman Empire in AD 476.

The Middle Ages (476-1453)

Until 1414, communion was administered in the Western Church in the two forms of bread and wine. That is why it was necessary to maintain a significant production of wine. Various invasions upset the cultivation of the vine, even though the majority of invading Burgundians and Visigoths spared the vine because they were superstitious – they were afraid of the magical powers of the monks and clergy who cared for the vines. The same situation arose during the Viking invasions in the ninth century AD.

The priests in the abbeys or the monks in the monasteries, who often became the great figures of Christianity, such as Saint Vincent, Saint Benedict and Saint Germain, encouraged the cultivation of vineyards by the clergy. In the Rule of Saint Benedict, it was laid down that it was sufficient for the monks to drink a quarter of a litre of wine each day. If a larger quantity was necessary, it "behoves the abbot to decide, taking care that there is no excess or drunkenness, since wine can cause even the wise to stumble".

In effect, it was preferable for a man of the Church to achieve spiritual ecstasy by fasting and prayer, rather than by drinking too much wine. However, Saint Benedict added: "It is better to take a little wine out of necessity, rather than a lot of water out of greed." During this period, wine was thus a part of the monastic ordinary. Monks had the right to a quarter of a litre of wine per day, except on feast days when there was no restriction. The rule was in fact quite generous because there were at least 150 feast days each year. However, though the Benedictine Rule was quite lax, there were other orders like the Cistercians who preferred to cultivate asceticism rather than the vine.

In AD 816, the Council of Aix-la-Chapelle gave a fillip to vine cultivation by encouraging ecclesiastical viticulture. Each bishopric had to have a "chapter" of canons responsible for cultivating vineyards and making them prosper. The cultivation of vines made a considerable jump forward during this period, since the clergy made up a fifth of the total population.

After Saint Bruno founded the Carthusian order in 1084, it was the turn of the former Cistercian Saint Bernard to set up his order at Clairvaux in 1153. All these monastic orders contributed to the development of wine growing in France. In the fourteenth century, wine had come to occupy such a position of importance in the life of the Church that the popes in Avignon even decided, as Petrarch reports, to make wine the fifth element to accompany air, water, fire and earth.

It was in this way, over the course of the centuries, that the men of the Church came to be the greatest growers and promoters of wine. This is not surprising because the demands on the resources of the Church were considerable: not only did the Church need to fulfil the need for wine at the Mass, but it had to cater for the pilgrims and travellers receiving hospitality in the monasteries, as well as the significant demands made on wine for medicinal purposes. For after all, this was a period when wine came to be used in many treatments and remedies. And then, of course, well protected palaces of the bishops were the obvious places for kings, emperors and princes to take a rest whilst on their journeys. And so the wine of the monasteries came to honour the tables of more prestigious hostels in the area.

With Charlemagne in the ninth century, princely viticulture was added to the ecclesiastical. A little later, at the beginning of the thirteenth century, Philip II of France even created a wine competition and presided over the main jury when circumstances would allow. In his book *The Battle of the Wines*, Henri d'Andeli reports that the prestige wines fit for the powerful were white wines. The most famous of these at that time, were the white wines from Beaune. As far as the wine from Argenteuil was concerned, it was judged "the most worthy for its goodness and its power to make even the King of France drunk". However, at court, sweet wines from Cyprus or Malaga were also appreciated. The peasant on the other hand still drank inferior wine from the second pressing, or again, vinegar cut with water.

As we might expect, in Paris where there were more than 4,000 taverns during the fourteenth century, a lot of wine was drunk. The huge demand gave rise to all sorts of fraudulent transactions, like cutting wine with water and colouring light red wines with blackberry juice. Only the noble and rich could obtain quality wines, which were normally served at the beginning and at the end of a mea, when homages were paid in the fashion of modern day toasts.

Wine was drunk from a shared cup passed around the assembled gathering. Goblets and individual glasses did not appear until the end of the fourteenth century, though the ceremony of drinking from a common cup continued until the seventeenth century. During the meal itself, where the dishes were preferably salty and spiced, water was normally drunk. It was after the evening meal having retired to one's room, that wine and pastries were consumed.

During this period, as in those that had gone before, spiced wines were very popular: these included *Clareia* (white wine, honey and cayenne), *Nectar* (white wine, honey, ginger and cinnamon), *Salviacum* (light red wine and sage) and *Hypocras* (wine from Beaune, sugar, cinnamon, ginger, cloves and nutmeg).

Concern with the quality of wine continued to develop. This is why in

1395 Philip the Bold, Duke of Burgundy, ordered the destruction of "the very bad and disloyal Gamay plant, for it is full of a great and horrible bitterness". However, it would seem that not a lot of attention was paid to his declaration, since it was renewed in 1441 by Philip the Good and again in 1486 by Charles VII.

From the fifteenth to the seventeenth century

During this period, wine was to cross a new frontier with regard to quality. Oenology, or the science and study of wines, makes its appearance and this new science was to result in much progress, particularly in the production of wine. The processes of sterilising and sulphuring the wine casks were refined using Dutch matches. Arresting fermentation in this way and evolving the technique of clarifying wine using egg white enabled wine to travel better.

But these developments only applied to top quality wines, since only the privileged could appreciate the improvements. Most of the wine produced remained mediocre, particularly as demand could not be satisfied. Production was about 72 litres per person per year, whereas consumption in the cities exceeded 107 litres per person. Those in the towns complained about the inevitable lack of wine which, moreover, gave rise to dues, taxes, tolls and other levies – all of which helped to make poor wines very expensive.

What sorts of wines were made during this period? Firstly, there were white wines. These came from grapes that were pressed by foot in vats, since the small producers wanted to avoid the costly business of having their grapes pressed in the vat belonging to the lord of the manor. The fermentation of the must was then completed in about 15 days, in a barrel with the bunghole left open. These were the ordinary, thick wines that were drunk with water, ice or perhaps snow. The practice of cutting wine with water, which surprises us today, was still the norm for the period. So much so in fact, that Furetières said in 1690 "only drunkards do not mix water with their wine!".

The famous light red wine called "clairet", made with a mixture of white and black grapes, represented about four-fifths of the wine drunk by the middle classes. The must derived from the rudimentary treading of the bunches of grapes was kept in the vats for two days, then the rose coloured liquid was transferred to a barrel where it continued to ferment. There was no pressing.

Ruby wine (the term "red" did not appear until the end of the eighteenth century) was obtained by pressing the grapes and leaving the mixture in the vats for longer and with a higher proportion of juice from the pressing.

Black wines were used for mixing with pale red wines that were too pale. They were drunk mainly by manual labourers. There was also a "vin de repasse" – the coloured water derived from flushing out the vats when they were emptied. This was the daily tipple of domestics and poor wine growers.

The inventory compiled by a taverner of the eighteenth century reveals the following distribution of wines: 38% ruby wines, 36% light red wines, 6% white wines and 2% cheap wines (*repasse* or coarse wines). Two-thirds of these wines were locally produced, but the producers were not normally specified.

The idea that wine was a food remained fundamental for the whole of this period. Gradually, however, a more hedonistic approach to wine developed. Coupled with a more refined style of life developing in the palaces, there evolved the concept of a wine also being drunk for pleasure. With the gradual development of gastronomy, the taste for great vintages appeared at the end of the seventeenth century. Black wines from the Bordeaux region were greatly appreciated by the English. Champagne, which had the reputation for making you feel exhilarated without making you drunk, invaded the court and worldly drawing rooms about this time. It enlivened the desserts and particularly amused the gathering when the cork popped and droplets of wine escaped into the generous *décolleté* of the pretty ladies present. As far as we know, Burgundies were already considered to be the great wines. They were specifically recommended by doctors, who prescribed them for their royal patients.

Unlike today, there was no problem about harmonising wines with their respective dishes, because the various dishes were placed "French Style" on the table at the beginning of the meal and the wines were placed on a sideboard and poured out on demand.

On the eve of the French Revolution, the nation barely totalled 27 million people. Ninety-two percent of the wine produced, including both top and medium qualities, was drunk by town dwellers who consumed on average, about 400 litres per year. At the king's palace at Versailles, average consumption was about 600 litres of wine per person per year and King Louis XIV was close to the top of the table.

However, if wine was not as widely available as the townsfolk would have liked, paradoxically it was more abundant than water. In Paris, for example, there were only 16 rather tired fountains supplying the whole city with water. It is difficult to imagine that there was more than a litre of water available per person per day. There were certainly aqueducts, but they only serviced Royal Palace, the homes of aristocrats, hospitals and convents.

The French Revolution

If the scarcity of bread incited revolt, then an additional cause for anger on the part of the people was that in Paris, wine too was becoming more and more scarce. It also became more expensive with the imposition of a local tax in 1790, enforced by 600 national guardsmen. In response to popular pressure, the National Assembly suppressed the tax on 19 February 1791 and red wine was bestowed with strong egalitarian, republican and brotherly credentials and was duly appointed the drink of the republican masses. With this it overthrew white wine, which had too many associations with the recently deposed head of state.

However, notwithstanding the good intentions of those in charge, as poverty became widespread in the towns, the effect of the revolution was to disorganise the supply of wine completely. In 1791, there were only 685 drinking outlets in Paris, as opposed to 4,000 in 1780.

Great wines which had been proscribed in conformity with the egalitarian principals of the Revolution, made their reappearance under the Directory after 1795, together with the Muscadins and the Incroyables[1], before gaining a place on the grand tables of Paris and eventually that of the Emperor.

1 *Muscadins and Incroyables* – Names given to the Royalists who distinguished themselves during the French Revolution by their foppish manners and dress.

The nineteenth century

When he published his *Almanach gourmand* in 1803, Grimod de la Reynière became perhaps the first gastronomic critic of modern times. He wrote: "According to many wine lovers, wine is man's best friend when used in moderation, and his worst enemy when taken in excess. It is our companion in life, a comforter in times of sorrow, an ornament to our prosperity, a fount of true feeling. It is the milk of the aged, the balm of adults and the ether of food lovers. The best meal without wine is like a ball without the orchestra." He extolled wine that was both natural and old, although he was aware that it was not easy to find in an age "where fraud and ignorance change into a dangerous poison, one of the sweetest presents of Providence".

The middle classes were great consumers of good wines. The enlightened wine lover of the nineteenth century was sufficiently refined to appreciate the variety of wines and to insist on quality. The hierarchy of "Grands Crus" from Bordeaux was institutionalised by the classification published before the Universal Exhibition of 1855.

But during the course of this century, as with those that went before, the same discriminations persisted: the peasant continued to drink *vinasse,* the close relation of vinegar, and the worker drank his coarse wine. We had to wait for 1868 before real wine – even if in small quantities – was given to the harvester to sustain him in his labours.

The middle classes used wine in cooking recipes; specialised terms evolved like *à la bourguignonne,* meaning "with red wine", *à la lyonnaise,* "with white wine and onions", *à l'alsacienne,* "with Riesling wine", *à la catalane,* "with Banyul wine, tomatoes, garlic, anchovies and cayenne", and *à la dieppoise,* "with white wine and cream".

The quality of wine continued to improve in the nineteenth century; thanks first of all, to the choice of grape varieties, but also the improvements to the vinification processes – particularly after the research on yeasts conducted by Pasteur. This research had been encouraged by Napoleon III, after the wines exported in 1863 proved to be undrinkable. Over five billion litres of wine were declared unfit for consumption and the French economy suffered a loss of more than five hundred million francs. Pasteur found the solution to the problem, which led to the publication of *Studies on wine, its diseases and their causes.*

New processes to keep wine and allow it to age. It is in this paper that Pasteur states that "wine is the healthiest and most hygienic of drinks".

The nineteenth century also saw great epidemics afflict the vine: pyrole caterpillar from 1828 to 1840; oidium from 1849 to 1857; phylloxera in 1870; mildew in 1878 and black-rot in 1885. After 1885, all the vineyards in France were reconstituted by hybridising plants and grafting French strains onto American stock which were found to be more resistant to disease.

However, if there was a lack of wine between 1879 and 1892 owing to the epidemics, over-production reappeared from 1893 to 1907. Legislation followed in 1894 to prohibit wine being watered down. The reduction of taxes and, above all, the coming of the railways were great stimuli to the sale of wine throughout France.

The twentieth century

At the beginning of the century, the production of wine in France exceeded consumption by 30%. In 1906, therefore, a law returned to home distillers the right to distil surpluses.

Unfortunately, however, these years of over-production did not discourage the activities of fraudsters; in 1907 the State took action against them. It compelled all wine growers to declare the size of their harvests and prohibited the addition of either sugar or water to wine. The anti-fraud service was created at the same time, as part of the Ministry of Agriculture. Fortunately the very bad wine harvest of 1910 allowed the wine surplus to be reabsorbed into the market and thus abate the anger of the wine growers.

Wine played a prominent role during the First World War. In the trenches, the *poilus*[2] called for wine. The army initially issued them with a quarter of a litre per day. Then twenty million litres of wine were offered by the wine growers in the south of France, which was quite a promotional coup at the time. After this, the army decided to buy 1.8 billion litres and to raise the soldier's ration to half a litre a day, without taking into account the tot given out before combat.

---

2 *Poilus* or "hairy ones" was the nickname given to the French soldiers in the First World War.

In 1916, after the victory at Verdun, the journalist-cum-writer Jean Richepin invited the French people to assemble on the field of battle with a glass of wine in their hands, so that the proceeds could then be given to the orphans and widows of France. In 1918, Marshal Pétain in his turn rendered a vibrant homage to wine "which has largely contributed to victory". In the meantime, the prohibition of absinthe (responsible for a great deal of alcoholism) further encouraged the increase in wine consumption.

But after the war, over-production reared its ugly head once more.

In 1930, the production of wine in the main body of France was 7.8 billion litres. To this was added a further 2 billion litres from Algeria, at a time when consumption in France was about 5 billion litres. To overcome this worrying over-production, new measures were introduced in 1931: a tax on production exceeding 10,000 litres per hectare (or one litre for every square metre), a ban on new planting and the distillation of excess production.

In 1931, a national council was set up to promote the drinking of wine. This increased the consumption of wine from 160 litres per person per year in 1905, to 172 litres per person per year in 1935. Gastronomy also made its contribution by developing a culinary literature based on wine. From the social angle, wine became a cultural phenomenon. It was in 1935 that the *Appellations d'Origine Contrôlée* (AOC) were introduced to protect specific production areas.

When the Second World War began, the soldier still received his ration of wine, though the satirical newspaper *Le Canard enchaîné* spread the rumour that the wine was adulterated with bromide and soldiers became very worried at the idea that they would be unable to fulfil their conjugal duties whilst on leave. Gradually, wine became increasingly rare – first for the soldiers, then for the civilians. In 1940, the situation became critical and wine was rationed at two litres per person per week. It should be added of course, that 60% of production in France went to Germany at this time.

After the Liberation in 1945, a new guarantee of wine quality was introduced – the *Vins Délimités de Qualité Supérieure* (VDQS). However, a new enemy appeared over the horizon in 1950: Coca Cola. Having already colonised the intellectual élite of Saint-Germain-des-Prés, the deputy Augustin Gros felt compelled to denounce the danger presented by this new drink imported from America. According to him, the product was toxic, full of phosphoric acid, caffeine and other substances that were impossible to identify since their formula remained secret.

Afraid of American colonialism and after a period of hesitation, the French Communist Party took up the campaign against Coca Cola on their own, and deputy Llante accused the national government of "allowing the stomach of the French to be poisoned". In a similar way, but with a little less aggression, the official commission for regulating the drinks industry in France, invited the government on 4 March 1950 "urgently to take the necessary measures to protect the interests of the national economy in general and agriculture in particular". In view of the size of the wine harvest the previous year and the difficulties associated with marketing it, on 7 January 1951 the municipal council of Beaucaire in the Gard even adopted unanimously a resolution calling for Coca Cola to be withdrawn from sale. This sort of protectionism, however, could not succeed and we all know how Europe finally succumbed to a brilliant marketing operation by the Americans.

In 1952, the Treaty of Rome inaugurated the European Community. However, it took almost 20 years before the common market for wine was finally introduced on 1 of June 1970. At first, intervention from Brussels consisted of acquiring a wine lake and then reducing it by distillation. Then in 1984, an agricultural policy was formulated based on the provisional programme adopted for table wines from the beginning of the wine growers campaign: in the case of over-production, distillation of the excess is immediate and obligatory.

And then, with the introduction of the Evin measure (a misnomer if ever there was one[3]) the last socialist government of Mitterand struck a further blow against the wine industry, when it drastically limited the scope for promoting wine in the French media. Not even the free circulation of goods within the Community is sufficient to guarantee the future survival of the industry in France.

It would seem that wine has begun its inexorable descent into the abyss, because consumption in France has continued to fall since the

---

3 The name *Evin* sounds like "et vin", meaning "and wine" – in the circumstances an unhappy play on words.

middle of the century: 62 litres per person per year in 1994, is exactly half the amount of wine drunk per person 40 years before. And the holders of the well-known Licence IV, which allows them to sell wine to all consumers, are disappearing as well. In 1910, there were 510,000 licensees catering for 38 million people; in 1992, there were barely 160,000 catering for a population of 58 million.

Bearing in mind this dramatic reduction in the amount of wine drunk, the future of French wine growers looks pretty sombre, for there is nothing to make one believe that their compatriots will not continue to steer clear of one of the finest flowerings of their national patrimony.

The situation is now all the more critical, as French wine growers are also confronted by competition from other European wine producers based in Italy and Spain. And with regard to exports, they have to compete with the expanding industries of California, Australia, New Zealand and even South Africa. In any event, for viticulture the years ahead will be decisive.

CHAPTER 3

FROM VINE BRANCH TO BOTTLE

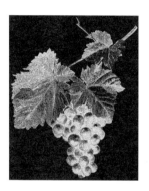

Wine is the product of the ground in which the vine is grown and the climate that prevails in a particular location. The interaction between these two factors, combined with the variety of vine grown and the skill of those who manage the vineyard, is what gives a particular wine its individual character.

THE GROUND OR "TERROIR"

The French word "terroir" conveys the concept of interaction and inter-dependence between the soil of a particular area and its climate, whether on a large scale like a region, or on a small scale like an individual slope. In English there is no exact equivalent of the French word. Various terms are used, but none incorporate all three ideas of soil, location and climate. The word "ground" seems as good as any.

The soil

The soil that lies near the surface of the earth has little importance for the vine. It is the nature of the ground beneath the surface that is the determining factor, for the roots of the vine stock penetrate well down into the rocky sub-soil to derive the mineral salts and trace elements that will nourish the plant.

Soils can be composed of silica, clay, limestone, sandstone, schist, granite or sand. Each of these rocks has a particular character that can give a unique quality to a wine. The presence of clay contributes to the colour and combination of tannins in a wine. Sandy soils are inclined to produce light wines that should be drunk when they are young. The reverse is true of schist and sandstone, which enable the wine to live longer.

In the same vineyard however, there can be a great variety of soils coming from different geological eras. In Alsace you find limestone, marls, sandstone, sands, granites and schist. In a geographical area like the Côtes de Nuits in Burgundy, there are more than 60 different types of soil.

The climate

The vine is sensitive to climate. It will grow well in temperate zones

47

between latitudes 30° and 50° North and latitudes 30° and 40° South. Planted anywhere else, the vine has difficulty in coping with the extremes of temperature.

The climate of a particular area may be considered in three different ways: the macro-climate typical of the region where the vineyard is to be found (Bordeaux, Burgundy, Moselle); the meso-climate, which is the local climate of the slope; and the micro-climate, which is the climate of a part of that slope.

The elements of a climate that have a significant effect on the vines are sunlight (particularly the amount received), temperature and the frequency with which it rains. A lack of sunshine, leading to ambient temperatures that are too low, will slow down the movement of sugar from the leaves to the grape. On the other hand, ambient temperatures that are too high will produce grapes lacking acidity.

In France there are four major wine growing areas, the product of four very specific macro-climates:

- areas with cool temperatures averaging 17°C, covering the Alsace, the Loire Valley and Burgundy

- warm temperate areas of the southwest and the Bordeaux region, where the average temperature varies between 17·5°C and 18·5°C

- warm temperate areas of the Côtes-du-Rhône and Provence with average temperatures between 18·5°C and 20°C

- warmer areas of the Languedoc-Roussillon and Corsica, with average temperatures between 20°C and 22°C.

The wind is also an important element, since it prevents the formation of grey mould by drying off the dew. It also accelerates the partial evaporation of water in the grapes, increasing their concentration of sugar.

The rainfall level is naturally of fundamental importance. The ideal amount is 400 to 600mm (16 to 24in) per year, spread evenly throughout the year, except during the final period of ripening from the middle of August to the wine harvest, when the rainfall should be as low as possible.

The air humidity (fog and mists) should also be low during the final phase of ripening, since it promotes the spread of grey mould, causing the grapes to burst, become too rich in acetic acid and have a musty taste. However, the formation of grey mould is actively encouraged in the production of sweet wines like Sauternes, to encourage *noble rot* as a part of the manufacturing process associated with a late harvest.

There are also other significant characteristics that relating to the local topography (elevation, plains, hills, slopes), for these have a particular effect on soil drainage.

THE VINE

The vine is in reality a creeper from the genus *Ampelopsis*, which also includes the Virginia creeper, and it is productive for about 75 years. These days we talk about old vines when they have been growing for more than 20 years. However, there are some very old vines – between 60 and 80 years old – that are still producing wine, often of exceptional though unfortunately limited quantity.

The different parts of the vine

- The "**Cep**" or **Stock** is the trunk of this small tree, which rarely exceeds a metre (3 ft) in height. It is often tortuous but quite decorative and so hard it can last a long time.

- The "**Sarment**" is the **Shoot** of the vine. It can vary in length depending on how it is pruned. It has therapeutic qualities and is often used as a tonic for the blood vessels.

- The "**Rafle**" is the woody part to which the individual grapes are attached. It grows out of the shoot.

- The "**Feuille de vigne**" or **Leaf** is attached to the shoot. This is the part of the plant that, through photosynthesis, produces the sugars that are stored in the grape.

- The "**Grain de raisin**" or **Grape** is covered by a skin which contains the aromas (terpenes) and polyphenols (antioxydants). These are the tannins, flavonoids of white grapes and the anthocyanines of red grapes, which will be dissolved during fermentation and eventually find their way into the wine. A coating of wax to which the yeasts attach themselves, covers the fine layer on the exterior of the grape – the cuticle that protects the grape from external attack. As we shall see, these indigenous yeasts (micro-organisms found in the environment) have a very important role to play in the subsequent fermentation of the grape juice.

The pulp of the grape is the moist part that contains the juice. As the grape matures, the composition of the pulp changes: the acidity decreases and the concentration of sugars increases.

The juice of the grape (must) is colourless, irrespective of whether the skin surrounding the grape is either green or black. In this state, its use is mainly as a diuretic and possibly a detoxicant.

The grape pips should not be crushed during pressing, because they will adversely affect the flavour and stability of the fermented grape. They can however be recovered and used to make an oil rich in polyunsaturated fatty acids (70%). However, the amount of oil produced is low, which makes it expensive.

Several of the constituent parts of the vine have therapeutic applications. The "vigne rouge" from the Bordeaux region, for example, is widely used in herbal medicines to treat problems associated with blood circulation (swollen legs, varicose veins, haemorrhoids), the menopause and migraine.

Vine stocks

The stock characterises the variety of the vine. Since the epidemics at the end of the last century (particularly phylloxera), there is no pure indigenous stock in Europe since all the vines had to be grafted on to American plants.

To have stocks that were more resistant to diseases such as oidum, mildew, black rot and phylloxera, a French scion was grafted onto American root-stock beneath the earth.

The choice of scion is crucial. There are two types available: one that is cloned or one that comes from seed. With cloned scion, all the cuttings come from the same plant – the mother stock – and from this, many identical daughter vines or clones are made. This technique, which is very productive, leads to a uniform collection of vines of medium quality. The second method gives rise to better quality vines, where each cutting comes from a different plant of the same variety in the same vineyard.

The *Institut National de la Recherche Agronomique* in Montpellier, has a complete collection of genetic material relating to the vine, thanks to uninterrupted work conducted by its researchers since 1876. The institute has 8,000 varieties of vine coming from 35 countries, from which they have derived 5,000 clones, 900 hybrids and 500 stock plants for grafting. Such a genetic reservoir is absolutely indispensable if we are to improve the variety of vines available.

The choice of grape varieties is very important, but these varieties must be appropriate for the soil and climate, for these condition the quality and character of the wine. This is the case, for example, with Pinot Noir in the Loire region, Cabernet-Sauvignon in the Graves and Médoc districts of the Bordeaux region, Syrah in the Rhône Valley or again Chardonnay on the chalky clay of the Côte-d'Or.

But the study and the choice of grape varieties is not only made in relation to quality or the land. It is also made according to the destination of the grape – whether the grape is destined for the table to be consumed as fresh or dried fruit, or whether it is destined to be processed into wine or maybe even distilled.

Principal White Grape Varieties

Chardonnay	Chasselas	Pinot Blanc
Chenin	Sylvaner	Gros Plant
Pinot Gris d'Alsace	Ugni Blanc	Romorantin
Sauvignon	Colombard	Roussanne
Gewurztraminer	Groset Petit Mauseng	Savaguin
Riesling	Marsanne	Viognier
Aligoté	Muscadet or Melon	

Principal Red Grape Varieties

Cabernet Franc	Syrah	Malbec or Côt
Carignan	Gamay	Mourvèdre
Pinot Noir	Cinsault	Merlot
Cabernet Sauvignon	Tannat	Negrette
César	Grenache	Pinot-Meunier

MAN

Wine is the fruit of the labours of both the wine grower and the expert, the oenologist. The former cultivates the vine and the latter cultivates the wine. Often these two roles are performed by one person.

The wine grower

His calendar is filled for the whole year. From October to March, the plants are at rest and the wine grower cuts the vine to limit the number of buds. In April, the buds open and everything is done to avoid damage caused by frosts. From April to June, growth is very strong and the branches that have grown out of old wood must be removed. In July, when the plants are in blossom, it is advisable to limit branch growth. August is the time to treat the plants once a week or fortnight against disease. In September, when the crop is fully ripened, it is time to harvest and the year has turned full circle.

At no time is watering encouraged, at least not in France; with American growers – particularly those in California – it is regular practice.

To produce good wine, scarcely any fertilizer is required. On the other hand, the vines should be kept well pruned and planted close together. If they are planted too far apart, the roots will stay too close to the surface and will not penetrate deep down to draw on the mineral salts which will give the wine the character associated with the ground in which it is grown.

Pruning also affects the quality of the wine. The more severe it is, the less watery and more concentrated is the wine. Even after a severe pruning, too many bunches may still develop. The wine grower will therefore thin out his crop during the month of July, thereby reducing the final size of his harvest to improve the quality of his wine. To compensate for the lack of humus in his soil, the grower may have recourse to fertilizer.

Adding fertilizer will dramatically increase the amount of wine produced, but it may be to the detriment of its quality. Contrary to what many believe, chemical fertilizers do not nourish the soil. Rather, they feed the plant. Meanwhile, too much potassium destroys the micro-flora and indigenous yeasts. In addition, it reduces the acidity of the earth. As a result, the level of acid in the wine has to be increased by adding tartaric acid. It is in this way that the chemical industry has become more and more indispensable to the wine grower: first, by supplying potassium as a fertilizer, then compensating by supplying tartaric acid, pesticides, herbicides, fungicides and chemical yeasts.

Fortunately, there are wine growers that are well aware of this situation and have returned to more traditional methods of raising their plants, using a form of organic farming. It is interesting to note that in France at the moment, 20% of the pesticides used containing copper and sulphur are applied to only 5% of the cultivated area. In addition, certain mushrooms have become resistant to fungicides, like *Botris cinerea,* which is responsible for grey mould that so terrorises the wine grower. The most effective treatments, used in the Champagne region in 1992, were only 20% effective. The cost effectiveness of such treatments being so low, it is hardly surprising that wine growers are seriously considering other ways of treating their crops.

The attitudes underlying the maxim "productivity is king and to hell with the consequences" are thankfully beginning to change. First of all, regulation has restored order in the majority of the *Appellations d'Origine Contrôlée*, by limiting the production authorised per unit land area. Also the market conditions are now quite different in France, where the consumption of cheap wine has declined considerably over recent decades. Only quality wines have a chance of surviving both in France and on the export market.

As far as harvesting the grape is concerned, there are now only two practicable methods. One is the traditional manual method, where the bunches are cut with secateurs, allowing the *rafle* or stalk to survive until the moment of pressing. The other is the modern method, where mechanical beaters separate the stalks from the grapes and then transfer them to the skip on a conveyor belt. This second method tends to damage the grapes and is not ideal for the production of wine from growths where the grapes should remain perfectly intact.

Organic wine growing

The concept of organic agriculture was born in France in 1932 and was reactivated during the 1960s. It was recognised in France with the legal directive of 4 July 1980, and later at the European level on 24 June 1991.

Three to seven years are required before land can be accepted as having been farmed organically, which is the time required for the residues of previous chemical treatments to disappear completely from the soil. In 1996, France had 106,108 hectares (262,193 acres) under organic cultivation, of which 4,738 hectares (11,708 acres) were dedicated to growing vines. These figures do not take into consideration land under-going conversion, and are spread over 15 administrative regions out of a total of 22.

Wine growing based on the principles of organic agriculture will help to rebuild a balanced ecosystem. Hedges planted to protect the vines from the wind will also shelter birds and insects. Rye and vetch sown between the rows of vines as a "green fertilizer" will shelter insects and micro-organisms that will help the vine to thrive. In addition, this "green fertilizer" will add composts that will stimulate biological activity in the soil.

Organic wine growing brings with it specific activities each season. In winter, the cuttings that come from the pruning, are buried with rock powder and marine algae to make a compost to fertilise the soil with humus and trace elements, without creating too much nitrogen, and this is the preferred way of both preventing disease and nourishing the vine. In spring, the topsoil is worked to aerate it and give it the suppleness it requires. The removal of old branches is done naturally by hand and in summer, even if the organically grown vines are less prone

Organic wine production – by region

Cl.	Region	Hectares	Acres
1	Languedoc-Rousillon	1628	4023
2	Aquitaine	1100	2718
3	Provence	905	2236
4	Rhône-Alpes	247	610
5	Burgundy	207	511
6	Centre	130	321
7	Poitou-Charente	105	259
8	Loire	202	499
9	South-Pyrenees	71	175
10	Corsica	55	136
11	Alsace	37	91
12	Champagne	27	67
13	Franche-Comté	15	37
14	Auvergne	7	17
15	Lorraine	2	5
	TOTAL	4738	11705

(Source: Revue du Sol à la Table)

to disease, treatment with mineral fungicides of sulphur and copper is still a necessity.

The organic wine grower brings considerable care to bear upon the task of disease prevention: proper ventilation of the grape by careful training of branches and selective removal of leaves. In the struggle against parasites which attack the grape clusters, he uses natural and not chemical methods. In autumn, the harvest is only conducted when the grapes have reached full maturity and only those grapes that are healthy and undamaged are taken to the winery for processing.

Organic wine production – by department

Cl.	Department	Hectares	Acres
1	Gironde	920	2273
2	Aude	531	1312
3	Hérault	630	1557
4	Gard	451	1114
5	Bouches-du-Rhône	352	870
6	Vaucluse	301	744
7	Dordogne	180	445
8	Var	155	383
9	Drôme	150	371
10	Côte d'Or	80	198
	TOTAL	3750	9267

(Source: Revue du Sol à la Table)

Organic wines

Subject to the same European regulation as organic farming, organic wine growing should try to use the "living forces" of nature to the full. Apart from using composts and hoeing, the organic wine grower should use homeopathic doses of preparations derived from plants: valerian (rich in phosphorus), horsetail (rich in silica), stinging nettles (rich in nitrogen) and dandelion among others. He should try to respect the lunar calendar when carrying out the different tasks associated with the vine (pruning, ploughing and handling) so as to limit the use of pesticides as much as possible.

This is the way that Nicolas Joly de Savennières has been cultivating his vineyard in the Maine-et-Loire for the last ten years, using neither pesticide nor insecticide. As a result, in 1991 he won the *Coulée de Serrant* presented by the gastronomic magazine Gault-Millau, "for one of the greatest dry wines of the world".

The oenologist

The wine grower of former times was also a sort of empirical oenologist, though he would have been surprised if he had been given that title, for with many years of experience behind him, he justly considered himself an expert in making wines. However, this is the specific task of oenology, since it is but the science of conserving and working wine in order to achieve optimum results.

Today, this work has devolved to the oenologist, whom we could consider a chemical engineer as a result of the specific training he has received. In effect, within a few decades, we have passed from the alchemist working in the wine storehouse to the specialised chemist working in his laboratory. The former placed his trust in the subtle perceptions of his nose, in his intuition as a man wedded to the land, in his sound peasant common sense and in the knowledge handed down to him by his ancestors. For after all, had he not been born as it is commonly said in the country "with his arse in the barrel"? The latter refers these days both to his senses and to his scientific knowledge, but above all to his sophisticated equipment for analysing and testing, as well as his computer.

In view of the fact that wine is as good today as it was in years gone by – some would say, even better – there is certainly no need to be nostalgic about the past.

Wine making

Grape juice is a spontaneous seat of fermentation. In the open air, this fermentation is acetic and gives rise to a sort of vinegar. In a closed vessel, the fermentation is alcoholic. It is the first step towards producing wine.

According to the accepted definition in Brussels for the European Community, "wine is a product obtained exclusively by alcoholic fermentation (either total or partial) of trampled or not trampled fresh grapes (or grape must) destined for direct human consumption".

The preparation of wine (as opposed to its "manufacture") is accomplished in controlled stages. Depending on whether one wants a wine to be red, rosé or white (dry or sweet) – or a sparkling wine using the champagne method – the techniques are different.

Without going into too much detail, let us examine how red wine is made.

The individual grapes or bunches are tipped into a fermentation vat and then crushed. The mixture of colourless juice and red grape skins is allowed to stand, so that the coloured pigments may dissolve. At the same time alcoholic fermentation begins, due to the action of microscopic mushrooms, called yeasts. These are attached quite naturally to the skin of the grapes as they are maturing. Over 300 varieties are known, but only a dozen are involved in the process of making wine. Fermentation ceases when all the sugars have been transformed into alcohol or when alcohol reaches a certain concentration.

The must (the mixture of pulp juice and pips) is left in the vats for a certain number of days, in a temperature that should lie between 28° and 32°C (82° and 90°F).

When fermentation is complete, the solid part of the mixture (the marc) is separated from the liquid part. This wine, called "vin de goutte", is of prime quality. The wine obtained by pressing the marc is of lower quality, called the "vin de presse". The two wines then undergo a second fermentation, called malolactic, which is indispensable for red wines. This will have the effect of lowering the acid level in the wine, by transforming the malic acid into lactic acid, which is only half as acidic.

During the wine making process, some corrections may need to be made. If the grape juice is lacking sugar, some will have to be added. This is called "chaptalisation". If the must is too acid, the level can be reduced by adding calcium carbonate or potassium bicarbonate. And then finally, if the grape is not acid enough, tartaric acid.

Chaptalisation is necessary in certain regions where there is not enough sunshine to produce the required concentration of sugar in the grape. Adding 1.7 kg (3¾ lbs) of sugar per 100 litres (26½ gallons) will raise the alcohol level in the wine by 1°. A moderate amount of chaptalising is acceptable and perfectly legal; it is quite another thing when it is done to excess, as unfortunately is so often the case.

In an "industrialised" vineyard, where the vines are treated with many different chemicals, the wild yeasts are often largely destroyed. The producer then has to use industrial yeasts, often selecting those that produce a lot of alcohol. The problem is that using standardised yeasts results in wines with a fairly uniform flavour. What is gained in terms of reliability is then lost in terms of character. Moreover, before industrial yeasting the must is treated with sulphur that inhibits the yeast and introduces complex aromas.

However, when left to its own devices, the land creates a microflora which evolves from one year to the next, according to the climate. It is this microflora which is responsible for the organic character of the wine, the taste and the nose, giving it the complex aromas which will help to type it.

Sulphur is used before, during and after alcoholic fermentation. It can even be added while the wine is being stored in the cellar. Sulphur is interesting for its anti-oxidising, anti-bacterial and anti-fungal properties. It improves the lasting qualities of wine and would seem to be indispensable for red wines that will be laid down for a long time. This is the reason organic wines that do not contain it tend not to age so well.

On the other hand, an excess of sulphites in white wines will tend to lead to headaches. In certain circumstances, it can be much more dangerous: quite recently, a German died from an asthmatic seizure after drinking a white wine high in sulphites.

The maximum amount of sulphites currently allowed by European Union is 160 milligrams per litre for red wines, 210 milligrams per litre for dry white wines and rosés, and 210 to 400 milligrams per litre for sweet wines containing 5 grams or more of sugar per litre. These maximum levels should be revised downwards before long.

Wine maturation

Once out of the vat made of stainless steel, concrete or wood, wine has to undergo several delicate processes that demand all the skill, intuition and tender care at the disposal of the oenologist. The different stages it will have to go through after it has been made into wine, are as follows:

- "**Soutirage**" or **Racking** which consists of transferring the wine from one container to the other. This process helps to clarify the wine by eliminating the lees or dregs and carbon dioxide.

- **"Filtration"** or **Filtering** which is done by passing the wine through fine membranes to clarify it still further.

- **"Ouillage"** or **Ullage**, which consists of topping up the vat or barrel to compensate for evaporation and absorption by the wood. It is done to stop air getting into the container and turning the wine into vinegar.

- **"Collage"** or **Fining**, which is the process of clarifying the wine by adding egg white, which combines with the particles in suspension causing them to sink to the bottom of the container. Gelatine, fish glue, casein or flocculous clay can be used instead of egg white.

- **"Stabilisation"**, which is the process that aims to stabilise the micro-organisms and the tartar in wine, to prevent the wine degrading in the bottle.

- **"Embouteillage"** or **Bottling**, which is followed by ageing in a cellar at a temperature between 10° and 12°C (50° to 54°F) and a humidity of 70%.

Nowadays, oenologists are divided into two categories: those called "stylists", who try to optimise the qualities of the wine by building on its personality derived from the ground on which it is grown; and those called "interventionists", who try to impose their own personality on the wine. The wine produced by the latter is no less worthy than that produced by the former, but it lacks the character of the place where it originated. When trying these wines, expert wine tasters recognise the oenologist more easily than the original vineyard.

Organic wines

These are, of course, wines that have been produced by wine growers using organic principles of cultivation. For a long time they have suffered the condescension of conventional wine growers and traders. Little by little they have succeeded in surprising and establishing themselves in the trade by producing some very good wines – even exceptional wines. As time goes by, they will become more and more a force to contend with.

In France at present, there are no more than 400 organic wine growers, producing 26 million litres (6,870,500 gallons) of wine per year – about 5% of French production in 1993. Among them are some prestigious names from the *Appellations Controlées* of Vosne-Romanée, Bonnezeaux, Chaume, Grand cru de Saint-Emilion, Nuits-Saint-Georges.

These wines are clearly healthier and of great quality. They are increasingly in demand, both in France and abroad, and their share of the market is therefore expanding very rapidly.

THE CONSUMPTION OF WINE

Over the last 40 years, the pattern of wine consumption has changed quite radically. Consumption in producing countries has dropped, particularly in France, whilst in countries where little or no wine is produced, consumption has gone up.

Consumption in France

Since the middle of the last century, France has kept records of annual wine consumption and this enables us to see how things have developed since that time:

Year	Litres/Person/Year	Year	Litres/Person/Year
1850	59	1960	129
1870	65	1980	91
1883	130	1988	85
1909	125	1990	74
1910	170	1992	64
1950	150	1994	62
1957	135	1995	65

(Sources: Boulet – INRA 1993 and OIV 1996)

Distribution of Occasional and Regular Wine Drinkers in France as a Percentage of their respective age groups

Age in Years	1980	1985	1990	1995
< 10	3.0	1.2	0.8	0.3
10–14	11.3	4.3	3.3	2.0
15–19	36.3	18.0	20.0	18.8
20–24	70.3	55.4	43.7	47.1
25–29	82.5	75.3	64.9	61.1
30–34	85.3	79.2	71.2	73.3
35–39	86.8	80.9	75.9	72.8
40–44	86.0	83.2	76.7	76.5
45–49	83.1	78.8	74.7	79.0
50–54	84.0	77.8	74.4	74.8
55–59	82.1	80.0	73.6	74.9
60–64	83.3.	73.8	70.9	75.8
65–69	79.5	74.0	74.2	71.6
70–74	76.7	72.9	70.4	76.4
>75	77.5	71.8	67.8	69.0
Average	76.4	69.9	63.8	65.3

(Sources: OIV 1997)

From the first set of figures we can see that in France, consumption went up by almost 290% between 1850 and 1910, and that from the end of the First World War until now, it has dropped by 60%. From the second set we can see that the major decline in wine drinking between 1980 and 1995, has been with the younger age groups. Wine drinking among those under 14 is virtually non existent and among those aged between 15 and 30, it has declined by about 20%.

Wine consumption among people over the age of 14

In France between 1980 and 1995, the percentage of regular or occasional wine drinkers has fallen from 76% to 65%, and the number of adults who do not drink wine has fallen from 24% to 35%.

Though it is not likely to surprise anyone, reference to the table below will show that there are more women than men who do not drink. There are two explanations for this. One is sociological: drinking alcohol is a male pastime. Peer pressure to drink wine is virtually non-existent for a woman although is very pronounced for a man. The other explanation is physiological: women have a lower tolerance to alcohol.

Wine consumption – combined figures for men and women over 15 years of age

Frequency	1980	1995
Every day	41.05%	22.8%
Almost every day	5.9%	5.0%
Regularly	46.9%	27.8%
Once or twice a week	10.9%	15.6%
Less frequently	18.6%	21.9%
Occasionally	29.5%	37.5%
All drinkers mixed together	76.4%	65.3%
Non-drinkers	23.6%	34.7%

(Source: Survey by INRA – Montpellier; ONIVINS)

Wine Consumption– the difference between men and women over 15 years of age

	Men		Women	
Frequency	1980	1995	1980	1995
Almost every or Every day	61%	37%	34%	18%
Once or Twice a week	10%	22%	12%	15%
Less than once a week	13%	18%	23%	22%
Never	16%	23%	31%	45%

With people over the age of 65, it has been observed that the older they become, the less wine they drink.

Wine Consumption– people over 65 years of age   (Department of the Lower Rhine)

Age	Men	Women
65-69	19.5%	1.0%
70-74	18.5%	1.2%
75-79	17.5%	1.2%
80-84	17.0%	1.2%
85+	11.0%	1.5%

(Source: Pradignac 1993)

Wine and the domestic budget

Since 1950, the amount of money spent by the French on wine as a proportion of what they spend on food has declined substantially. In 1992, purchases of wine accounted for 10% of what was spent on food. This is a negligible amount of money, but the decrease in volume of wine drunk has been greater than the statistics would indicate, because people are drinking less and less of the cheaper table wines.

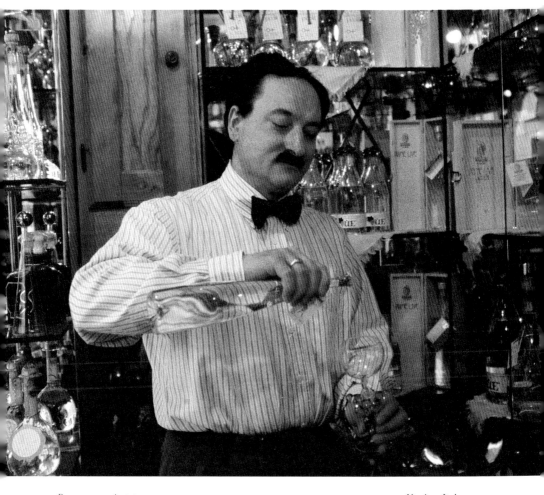

Barman pouring grappa.   *Venice, Italy.*

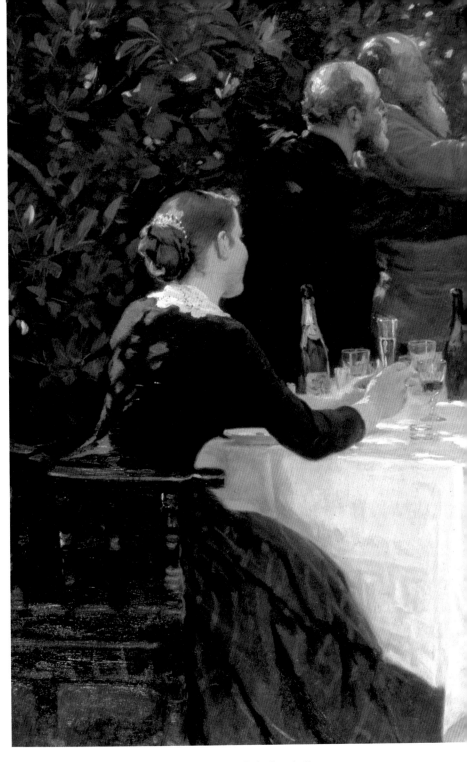

"Party in the garden of the artist", (Skagen, 1888). By Peder Severin Krøyer.

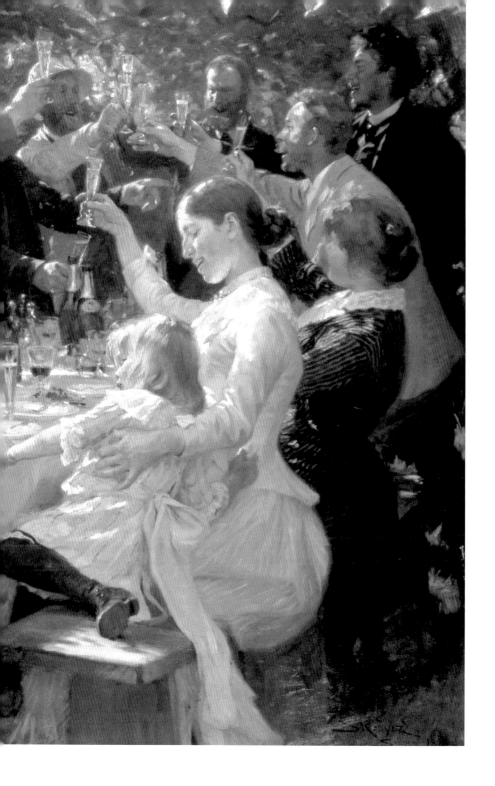

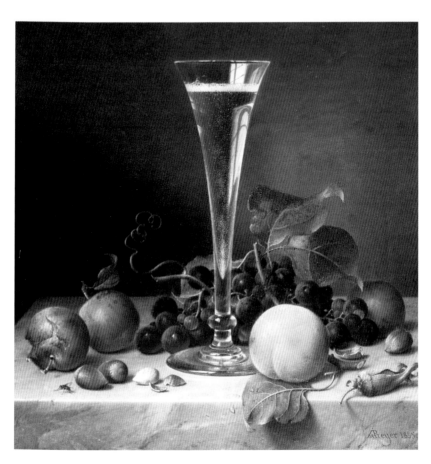

"Champagne with fruit" by Preyer Johann Wilhelm.

Consumption of Table Wines in France   **(Average per person per year)**

Year	Litres
1955	128
1960	120
1970	100
1980	85
1985	65
1990	45
1995	30

(Source: INSEE 1996)

Instead, French people are drinking more and more quality wine. However, this consumption is mainly associated with festive occasions, so the total amount of wine drunk has declined quite substantially over recent decades.

Consumption of Quality Wine in France

Frequency	1980	1992
Each day	9%	23%
Festive occasions	35%	38%
Entertaining guests	48%	71%

(Source: OIV)

Even if these statistics are fairly reassuring, they show that 29% of the French do not place a quality wine on the table when they have guests. Which shows that there is plenty of room for improvement in a country that considers itself one of the major wine producing countries in the world.

Geographic distribution of wine drinkers in France

The majority of French people drink wine because it is part of their culture. And yet, from one region to another, from one department to another, the average consumption of wine can double. Who would have thought Burgundy would have the lowest average of 25% and that Picardy, where vines are as rare as coconut trees, would have the highest of 46%?

Most unexpected is the discovery that the most rapidly shrinking group of wine drinkers, is the one whose members drink wine on a regular basis: many of these people are now joining the ranks of those who only drink wine from time to time. In the Ile-de-France, which includes Paris, in the Champagne region, in the North, in Normandy, Picardy and Franche-Comté, only a quarter of the population drink wine regularly. Among these regions, the decline is most pronounced in the Ile-de-France, in the North and Northeast.

Why do the French drink less wine?

It is interesting to analyse the reason why there are French people who drink no wine at all and why there are others who no longer drink wine on a regular basis. It is also surprising to learn that both groups are expanding all the time.

Wine Consumption – reasons for abstaining

Principal Reason	1990	1995
"I do not like the taste"	53.1%	61.7%
Hygienic or health reasons	27.3%	17.4%
No alcohol as a matter of principle	13.8%	5.8%
"Those around me do not drink"	4.6%	3.3%
"I have never had the opportunity to appreciate wine"	2.3%	2.3%
Influenced by anti-alcohol lobby	1.2%	1.6%
Gives a bad image of oneself	0.5%	0.7%
Too expensive	0.4%	0.4%
Other reasons	6.8%	6.8%

Wine Consumption – reasons for not drinking regularly

Principal Reason	1990	1995
"I do not think about it"	18.5%	20.7%
"I have no need"	32.5%	29.4%
"I reserve it for special occasions"	26.8%	22.8%
"Those around me do not drink regularly"	8.2%	3.4%
"It is not compatible with my work"	4.5%	1.8%
Influenced by advice to limit drinking	0.9%	15.9%
Too expensive	3.0%	1.5%
Other reasons	5.6%	4.5%

(Source: INRA ONIVINS)

An examination of these two tables reveals that the number of people who do not actively like the taste of wine, has increased from 53.1% in 1990 to 61.7% in 1995. This is very much the product of culture and education and unless we make a conscious effort to hand on our heritage of wine, it will be replaced by other drinks that are promoted by specific commercial interests, which have nothing to offer other than an image created by media experts.

It is quite striking how the proportion of people not drinking wine for health reasons has gone down by 10% – which does at least show that the French are aware that drinking wine is compatible with good health. However, it is clear that campaigns aimed at reducing alcoholic intake have been successful in causing many people who formerly were regular drinkers into becoming occasional drinkers (+15% in 5 years).

Future perspectives

French wine growers have been fortunate. Some are rich because their vineyard is well-known. Others are less so. But altogether, it is a profession that has acquitted itself with honour, particularly as wholesale prices have increased very little over the last ten years. However, what the future holds for French wine grower ten or twenty years from now, when the consumption by their fellow citizens continues to decline as it has done in recent years, nobody can tell.

If this decline in consumption continues at its present rate, pessimists will tell us that the French will no longer be drinking any wine by the year 2010! Optimists believe on the other hand, that traditional cultural patterns will ensure this does not happen. They cannot believe that the proportion of wine-drinking Frenchmen could conceivably drop below 50% by the year 2000.

This is the reason professionals who refuse to adopt a pessimistic view of the future maintain that with the beginning of the third millennium, the wine-drinking population of France should be made up as follows: 25% to 30% regular drinkers, 39% to 41% occasional drinkers and 30% to 40% non-drinkers.

To summarise then, we might define the "new" wine-drinking Frenchman in the following way: he will drink less but better wine (little or no "vin ordinaire"); he will be more of a wine connoisseur but will be less regular in his drinking habits.

This means that in the years to come, wine growers will only be successful if they pay due attention not only to the quality of their wines but also to the quality of their public relations.

Global trends in the consumption of wine

This apparent aversion to wine is not specifically a French problem. It affects all the wine producing countries, though it is interesting to note that wine consumption has increased in non-wine producing countries.

Consumption in litres per person per year

Country of Production	1975	1990
Italy	110	70
Portugal	90	85
Spain	75	48
Greece	37	35

(Source: OIV)

Consumption in litres per person per year

Non-producing Country	1975	1990
Great Britain	4	10
Denmark	10	30
Netherlands	10	14
Belgium	16	19
Germany	22	26
Japan	0	1.2

(Source: OIV)

Germany has been included in the list of non-producers in spite of the fact that it has a wine producing region in the Southwest (Moselle). However, as a country it has always been a weak consumer: a third of its production is exported to the USA and to the European Community.

Nonetheless, French wine producers can take heart from the opportunities offered by exporting their wines into those countries that do not produce wine, where consumption continues to rise whilst that in France seems to be in permanent decline [1].

1 See Appendix 2, Table 1 for complementary statistics on wine consumption in the principal countries of the West.

CHAPTER 4

WINE IS A FOOD

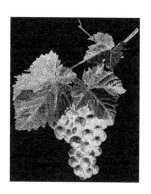

Food is a nourishing substance containing macro- and micronutrients which contribute to the nutritional needs of the human organism. In the light of this definition, wine is without doubt a food because it contains macronutrients (carbohydrates, some proteins) that give energy, and above all it contains micronutrients (mineral salts, trace elements and even vitamins).

The nutritional value of a food is normally expressed in terms of its chemical composition per 100 grams. For a drink, the composition is given for a 100 millilitres of liquid, or alternatively 1 litre, which is ten times as much. For wine, it is more convenient to conduct the analysis in terms of a litre, which can then be easily divided by 2 or by 3 to give doses that can reasonably be consumed each day.

THE NUTRITIONAL COMPOSITION OF WINE

Proteins

There are very few proteins in wine: about 1or 2 grams per litre. However, although they are present in very small quantities, almost all the essential amino acids are there, as well as some peptides – which are molecules made up of several amino acids.

This lack of protein in wine, particularly when compared to grape juice, is due in part to the fining process that causes the wine to throw a sediment. In these solids that precipitate to the bottom of the barrel, are to be found many of the proteins originally present in the grape juice

Since the daily intake of protein should be at least 1g/kg (1 gram per kilo of body weight), wine would not therefore classify as being an exceptional source.

Carbohydrates

Alcoholic fermentation transforms the greater part of the grape juice sugars into alcohol, thanks to the action of the yeasts in the must.

In red wine, the residual sugars (glucose and fructose) are not very important (about 2 or 3 grams per litre). In white wines, they can be more important: up to 20 g/l (20 grams per litre) for some very fruity wines, and 100 g/l for certain very sweet wines. We know that the association of sugar and alcohol is not desirable, as it leads to hypoglycaemia.

In addition to carbohydrates, wine also contains other sugars, such as polyols (alcohol sugars), glycerol or sorbitol.

Lipids or fats

Wine does not contain lipids. It is particularly important that none should be present when the wine is being processed, since they would adversely affect the taste. Care must be taken with the pips, however, as they could release oil when crushed.

What look like oily deposits on the side of an empty wineglass are in fact the products of complex carbohydrates combining with anthocyans (polyphenols).

Fibre

In food analysis tables, fibre is not shown as being a constituent part of wine. In reality various grape fibres such as pectin, are soluble and probably exist in wine in their liquid state. However, current methods for measuring fibre content are unable to detect fibre in wine.

Water

A litre of wine contains a variable amount of water: 730 ml for a sweet wine, 880 ml for a white wine with 11° of alcohol, 920 ml for a red wine with 12°.

Alcohol

In fact, it would be better to talk about "alcohols" since there are various types contained in wine. The proportion of alcohol is 75 g/l in a 9° wine, 88 g/l in a 11° wine, 96 g/l in a 12° wine and 102 g/l in a sweet wine. However, these are only average figures, since the degree of alcohol in a wine depends on the level of sugar in the grapes when they are harvested and whether they are chaptalised. It should also be borne in mind that the level of alcohol in a wine decreases with time.

Apart from ethyl alcohol, wine contains very low quantities of propylic, butylic and amylic alcohol. Fortunately, methylic alcohol (or methanol) only exists in minute quantities as it is very toxic. This is the reason wine growers are forbidden to plant vines that produce significant amounts of it; methanol is responsible for all sorts of side effects summed up in the word "hangover" – headaches, thirst, sweatiness, shaking, fatigue and nausea.

Mineral salts

Some, for example potassium, are present in significant quantities. We should remember that the concentration of these mineral salts should be divided by a factor of 2 or 3 in order for us to appreciate what is likely to be consumed each day.

Magnesium and calcium are ionised and therefore easily absorbed in the small intestine. Salt is present in such low quantities that even those on a salt-free diet can drink wine.

Mineral Salt	Concentration in one litre of wine	Recommended daily intake for an adult
Potassium	700 to 1,600 mg	2,000 to 5,000 mg
Calcium	50 to 200 mg	1,000 to 1,500 mg
Magnesium	50 to 200 mg	330 to 420 mg
Sodium	20 to 250 mg	2,000 to 4,000 mg
Phosphor	100 to 200 mg	1,000 to 1,500 mg

Trace elements

Certain wines – Médoc – are rich in iron. Moreover, the iron is ionized, which means it can be easily assimilated through the intestines.

Wine can therefore be an interesting source of iron, though too much tannin in the wine can interfere with its absorption through the wall of the intestines. On the other hand, wine may contain other trace elements that are less desirable than iron, like aluminium, lead and perhaps arsenic.

Since 1996, the level of lead in wine must not exceed 0.2 g/l. Its presence in the grape is due to the exhaust fumes emitted by cars that still run on leaded fuels and pollute the vines that run along the side of the road.

Trace element	Concentration in one litre of wine	Recommended daily intake for adults
Iron	2 to 10 mg	10 to 18 mg
Copper	0.2 to 1 mg	2 mg
Zinc	0,1 to 5 mg	12 to 15 mg
Manganese	0.5 to 3 mg	5 mg

Vitamins

Even if wine contains vitamins, the quantities are infinitesimal. In addition to this, vitamin B1 is rendered inactive by sulphites present in many wines, particularly cheap ones. We should also be aware of the fact that although present in the grape, in wine, vitamin C is totally absent and vitamin B12 is only present in minute quantities.

Vitamin	Concentration in one litre of wine	Recommended daily intake	
		Men	Women
B1 thiamine	0.1 mg	1.5 mg	1.3 mg
B2 riboflavin	0.1 to 0.2 mg	1.8 mg	1.5 mg
B3 niacin	0.7 to 0.9 mg	18.0 mg	15.0 mg
B5 pantothenic acid	0.3 to 0.5 mg	10.0 mg	10.0 mg
B6 pyridoxine	0.1 to 0.4 mg	2.2 mg	2.0 mg

Polyphenols

This is certainly one of the most interesting aspects of wine. The concentration of polyphenols goes from just a few milligrams in white wines to 1.2 g/l or even 3 g/l in red wines.

To start with, they are concentrated in the skin of the grape, in the pips and the stalk, and it is the alcohol that allows them to move into the wine. It is these anti-oxidants that give wine its power to inhibit cardio-vascular disease, as well as the growth of cancerous tumours and the development of Alzheimer's disease. However, we shall return to examine them at greater length in the next chapter.

There are various types of polyphenols – phenolic acid, flavonoids (or the vitamin factor P), anthocyans including tannins, flavonols like procyanidols and catechins, quinones, cumarins, and resveratrol.

Mineral acids

These are mainly tartaric, malic and salicylic acid. They contribute to make wine into a liquid alcoholic acid, with a pH between 2 and 3, which approximates very closely to that of the stomach. They therefore assist the digestion of alimentary protein, found particularly in meat.

Other substances

Wines also contain aldehydes (20 mg/l) which in conjunction with esters, alcohols and phenols, make up the volatile substances responsible for the aromas. But it is also possible to discover substances in wine which lead to problems, such as sulphites, histamine, tyramine and serotonin.

DOES WINE GIVE YOU ENERGY?

For centuries in France, wine has sustained manual workers in their efforts, because they believed it gave them energy. My great-great-grandfather had a forestry company in the second half of the nineteenth century. He was under contract with his men, who used to saw tree trunks into planks by hand, using a long saw, to supply them with four litres (1 gallon) of wine per day or 40 cl (more than ¾ pint) per hour of work. When this was added to what they drank at mealtimes, they drank 6 litres (1½ gallons) of wine a day. What is even more extraordinary is that several of them lived to what was considered in those days, a very respectable age.

Nearer to our times, in September 1949, a medical congress in Bordeaux concluded as follows: "A manual worker should drink more than a litre of wine per day and an intellectual should drink at least half-a-litre, in order for both to stay in good health."

However, scientific work done since does contradict this generally accepted idea, though it is hard to convince those who see wine with its 500 to 600 kcalories per litre, as quite an acceptable "fuel" for the body.

So let us see what happens to alcohol, the only energy-giving constituent of wine, once it has penetrated the body.

First of all, there is considerable heat loss. Everyone has noticed this phenomenon at "well-lubricated" dinners, when guests will remove their jackets given half a chance. By the same token, after drinking wine for supper, a blanket at bedtime is far less necessary, since 65 to 70% of the energy contained in alcohol will be dissipated as heat.

But this phenomenon is more obvious in the case of thin people than with fat people and it is more intense with those that are active than with those that are sedentary. This is why, if you take exercise like walking after having drunk alcohol with a meal, you will start to dissipate heat. This will ensure better bodily ventilation and suppress the disagreeable congestion you might have experienced by remaining inactive in a enclosed area.

About 5 to 10% of this energy will be discharged through the urine, sweat, and even vapour expelled from the lungs. Only 20% of the energy will go to the brain, nervous tissue and red blood cells. Contrary to what many have thought for a long time, this energy is not available for the muscles.

Finally, in the case of alcoholic excess, 5 to 10% of the energy will be transformed into fat to be stored in the liver (hepatic steatose).

WINE AND SPORT

More than a very modest intake of alcohol (that is, more than 2 glasses of wine), can become a severe handicap for the sportsman, owing to the adverse effects it has on the muscles.

When there is alcohol in the blood, the uptake of glucose (the proper fuel for the muscles) is reduced by 30%. In addition, the mechanism that normally allows the body to transform fat reserves into glucose when required, is blocked. There is also an increase in acidosis, which will limit endurance, and an increase in the accumulation of waste products from the metabolism, like urea and uric acid. Finally, in addition to the risk of hypoglycaemia, there is also the risk of losing magnesium through the urine.

So, contrary to what has been generally thought, an excess of alcohol can contribute to a change in muscular performance, with a reduction in tone and a lengthening of response time during an extended activity.

However, if a sportsman indulges in alcohol there can be additional penalties. The rapid movement of cellular water into general circulation can lead to a disturbing feeling of heaviness, particularly in the arms and legs. What is more, the increase in the amount of urine brought about by the diuretic effect of alcohol, will accelerate dehydration. In addition there is a slight contraction of the bronchial tubes which diminishes the oxygenation of the blood.

It is important for the sportsman to realise that the sensation of heat generated by drinking alcohol is very superficial. Paradoxically, there is a reduction in internal body temperature that will be all the more marked if there has been an inadequate intake of complex carbohydrates beforehand. This can help us understand the dangers inherent in having a coffee laced with alcohol or having a warm punch, either before or during physical activity conducted in the cold, like skiing, skating or climbing mountains. At the top level of sport, even the smallest amounts of alcohol will result in reduced performance.

To summarise then: taking alcohol before or during sporting events, will result in dehydration, a lack of glucose in the muscles, a reduction in performance and awareness which can easily lead to a severe accident.

And what happens when the sporting activity is over? In the aftermath of strenuous physical activity, it is imperative that the sportsman should be careful, particularly if the activity resumes the following day, as may happen with tennis competitions. Drinking alcohol after a major physical exertion can have the effect of increasing acidosis leading to tendonitis, interfering with muscular recovery after extended periods in fixed positions (cycle racing) and increasing the loss of mineral salts, which will prolong the effects of fatigue.

Regular alcohol excesses between competitions (particularly when engaged in team sports like rugby) can result in vitamin loss (vitamin B1 necessary for metabolising glucose or vitamin D for metabolising minerals necessary for healthy bones) and mineral loss (calcium or magnesium, leading to muscular cramp).

Sportswomen, who have half the quantity of alcohol-metabolising enzymes and less muscle mass, are particularly vulnerable to small daily doses of alcohol.

An athlete may drink a couple of glasses of wine during a meal (particularly at dinner) during rest periods or training, but not the day before, the day of the competition or the day after.

Taken in this way, wine will allow the sportsman to benefit from the powerful anti-oxidising effect of polyphenols, which combat the damaging action of free radicals. These are released in great numbers into the bodies of people engaged in top-level sport. It must be remembered however, that moderation is the name of the game, because an excess of alcohol will lead to an excess of free radicals.

Sport has a useful role to play in helping an alcoholic with his or her rehabilitation. Walking or cycling are particularly suitable. For those who want to engage in top-level sport, and are able to do so, the marathon or triathlon are excellent disciplines for developing will-power. As far as the martial arts are concerned, they can be of considerable benefit, particularly in view of the ideas and philosophical concepts they enshrine.

DOES WINE MAKE YOU FAT?

When they started drinking only water, men who were formerly quite substantial wine drinkers and overweight into the bargain, have noticed that they have lost several kilos in weight. On the other hand, there are men who claim to have had startling results when following Phase One of the Montignac Method, whilst continuing to drink the generous glass of wine they had resolved never to give up at the end of each meal. So, does wine make you fat?

However you look at it, wine is energy

Everyone knows that foods containing calories impart energy. One gram of protein contains 4 kcal, 1 g of carbohydrate contains 4 kcal and 1 g of fat contains 9 kcal. A gram of alcohol contains 7 kcal. The calorific value of wines vary according to the amount of alcohol and according to the amount of sugar they contain: 540 kcal for a litre of 9° red wine; 700 kcal for a litre of 11° white wine; 1520 kcal for a litre of sweet white wine.

Is knowing the calorific value of wine of any interest? It is after all a theoretical figure for wine in a bottle; once the wine has been consumed, its future is very variable. In fact, the absorption of calories varies according to the time of the day. In the evening it is more pronounced than it is in the morning. The use of calories is also very variable, depending on whether wine is consumed on an empty stomach or during the course of a meal (as can be easily determined on both occasions, from measurements of alcohol in the blood). And then, it depends on the type of meal that has been eaten, since the absorption of alcohol (like sugars) is more or less dependent on the quantity of fibre, particularly soluble fibres, contained in the food.

In addition, we now know that a diet low in calories is the best guarantee against slimming. For a long time, studies have shown that the energy factor is not decisive in causing people to gain weight. In order to slim, people should choose on the basis of quality and not on the quantity of food. The obsession with calories as a way of losing weight is now totally outmoded. It is therefore much more interesting to look into studies that have sought to determine whether the consumption of wine *encourages* weight gain or not, and in their light ask ourselves whether we can continue to drink wine if we want to lose weight.

Wine and diet

Let us start by saying that the statistics show the percentage of obese people who drink wine is no higher than the percentage of those that do not. Having said this, it is important to know that the effect of wine is not

81

linked to the number of glasses drunk, but to the importance this energy intake represents when compared to the meal with which it is associated.

If wine (say three or more glasses) is added to a normal meal, it can in fact contribute to weight gain. If on the other hand, it replaces food that would normally have been eaten, then not only will it not cause you to get fat, it could even help you to slim.

This comes back to saying that in replacing part of the energy from the meal, you will tend to slim. This is true, but is important to point out that this slimming when it does take place, will be at the expense of the non-fatty mass of the body. This could be dangerous. So everything depends on whether wine replaces the carbohydrates or the fats in the meal.

In any event, what is certain is that by drinking a glass of wine at the end of a meal, you will be contributing to the reduction of fatty mass in your body in two ways: firstly, by reducing the secretion of insulin (-1.4 units per litre of blood) and secondly, by increasing energy expenditure by 7%.

It has been noticed that older people do not absorb nutrients well through the intestinal wall and their reduced enzyme output will make it more difficult for them to store alcohol, by preventing its transformation into fats suitable for storage in the body. This leads us to conclude that excessive drinking is more easily tolerated by older people than it is by young adults.

In conclusion, we can say that up to 30 grams of alcohol per day – which is equivalent to three 10cl glasses of wine – taken in the middle of the two main meals of the day, will not cause a healthy person of average stoutness to put on weight (when on Phase 2 of the Montignac Method, for example).

For somebody trying to lose weight (Phase 1), this amount of alcohol can be consumed without risk of interrupting the slimming process, providing an equivalent amount of fat is removed from the daily diet.

For a man or woman with a very sedentary lifestyle who is trying to lose weight, the daily consumption of wine should be reduced to two glasses of wine a day, drunk at the end of each of the two main meals.

CHAPTER 5

Wine as a Medicine since Ancient Times

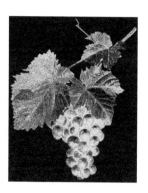

The history of medicine from ancient times has taught us that since its discovery by man, wine has featured prominently in his arsenal of healing aids.

Wine remained one of the most frequently used remedies in traditional medicine, from the times of the ancient Greeks, Egyptians and Romans, through biblical times, the Middle Ages, the Renaissance, the Age of the Enlightenment and the age that gave rise to the Industrial Revolution. It held this honourable position until modern biology replaced it with other medicines created by the pharmaceutical industry.

Stripped of its medicinal aura, wine became easy prey for the anti-alcohol lobby after the Second World War, when it was driven into the ghetto of suspect drinks.

In the last 25 years, eminent doctors, including Professors Masquelier and Renaud, have tried in vain to convince the world that this treatment of wine is unjust because modern scientific research actually confirms the many beneficial effects it has on health.

It needed the recent media coverage in the United States, on the now famous *The French Paradox* by Lewis Perdue, for the world to rediscover that wine is also a medicine and that it has exceptional medicinal properties with regard to the prevention of cardiovascular disease.

The oldest record of wine being used therapeutically is an inscription discovered by archaeologists in the tomb of Plah-Hotep, who is thought to have lived in Egypt about 4,000 BC. In addition, a similar message was found on a tablet in the Sumerian city of Nippur, which is thought to date from about 3,000 BC.

In Ancient Greece

In earliest times, the ancient Greeks practised incantatory medicine in their temples dedicated to Asclepios the god of health. But with the passage of time, this was replaced by the application of authentic remedies. Among these remedies, wine held a privileged position.

Homer tells us, for example, that Philocetes was wounded during the siege of Troy and, was cured with wine from Podaleirus. But it is with Hippocrates (460–377 BC) the father of modern medicine, whose many precepts are still relevant today, that wine was consecrated as the great healer. When taking their oath, modern doctors should bear in mind these words of the master: "Wine is a marvellously appropriate thing for man if in health as in illness, it is administered at the right time and in the right measure according to individual constitution."

Hippocrates, who was not without humour, maintained that austerity and sadness were responsible for illness. This is why he advised drinking wine, for he said "it expands the spleen and gives happiness". However, he did not advocate wine indiscriminately when he added: "things are only a cure when applied at the right time. Wine is a medicine if it is given at the right time: if on the contrary wine is administered at the wrong time so that it results in frenzy and delirium, it can no longer be called the remedy but rather the cause of illness."

But other than internal use, Hippocrates advised using wine in dressings or ointments, to treat wounds or certain forms of rheumatism. A little later, Theophrastes (372–287 BC) invented medicinal wines by mixing them with herbs and spices possessing well-known healing properties.

In Rome

In ancient Rome, wine lost none of its therapeutic properties. Numerous authors bear testimony to it.

In his treatise *De Materia Medica*, Dioscorides (first century AD) wrote: "Good natural wine warms, is easily digested, is good for the stomach, excites the appetite, is nourishing, improves sleep, fortifies the body and gives it a healthy colour."

Pliny the Elder, killed at Pompeii in 79 AD whilst satisfying his professional curiosity as a naturalist, recalled in his treatise on natural history the medicinal applications not only of wine, but also of the vine shoot, the vine leaf and the pips of the grape. He also mentioned that "Wine is a tonic, an aperitif, an hypnotic or a euphoric which improves the digestion" and agreeing with Hippocratic teaching, he confirmed that "Wine by itself is a remedy; it nourishes the blood of man, it gladdens the stomach and cushions both sadness and worry."

In his turn, Celsus – a doctor in the century of Augustus – confirmed the ideas of Galen concerning the beneficial influence of wine on the health of the person who uses it. And everything leads us to believe that the Romans of this period took pains to follow these wise counsels. Petronius for instance has left us an account of this famous banquet speech offered by Trimalcio, who addressed his guests in these terms: "wine lives longer than man: let us therefore drink like sponges, since wine is life". We can conclude by quoting Galen (130–201 AD), who recounts how he treated the troubled digestion of the emperor Marcus Aurelius: "I prescribed him a glass of wine sprinkled with pepper."

In biblical times

The Bible mentions wine 450 times for its beneficial effects. Thus Saint Paul suggests to Timothy that he should treat his stomach ulcer by drinking some wine. The Talmud of Babylon too, considered that wine was the most effective of medications.

In the Middle Ages

With the fall of the Roman Empire, the works of Hippocrates and Galen were temporarily forgotten. God was now considered the only source of healing for those who had faith. Only the monks of this period were wine growers, producing wine for use in the Mass and to care for their patients by mixing it with crushed herbs cultivated in their gardens.

But with the expansion during the ninth century of the School of Medicine at Salerno, in the Campagna south of Naples, the belief that wine held many therapeutic virtues began to resurface once again. So much so in fact, that over the main door of the hospital were engraved these words: "Drink a little wine".

The teaching books of this prestigious "faculty of medicine" spelt out this principle in even greater detail. "Good wine" they said, "revitalises the aged. Pure wine gives many benefits: it acts as a tonic for the brain, makes the stomach happy, chases away evil humours and clears the overloaded organs. It makes the mind agile, the eyes shiny, the ear more acute, does away with overweight and imparts to life robust health."

As well as the School of Salerno, which was very influential until the twelfth century, the famous Arab doctor Avicenna (980–1037) also extolled the merits of wine. He fervently maintained that it was "the best friend of a wise man".

Towards the end of the Middle Ages – namely during the twelfth, thirteenth and fourteenth centuries – scholastic medicine emerged with the establishment of faculties of medicine, like that at Montpellier in 1220. It was in these places of learning that ancient medical texts were dissected and used as sources of inspiration.

In the *Book of Antidotes* by Nicolas, almost half the medical "recipes" contain wine; and during this period, wine is more often than not one of the fundamental ingredients of a medicine. It is the period of the famous theriac, a potion for combating poisonous bites, which contained many ingredients including wine. All of these preparations aimed to "reconstitute the heat of the body", "unblock the vessels of the liver, spleen and bladder", get rid of "harmful humours", aid digestion or wash wounds. Their scope was vast, because many of the remedies containing wine were suited for external application.

Henri de Mondeville (1260–1320) a famous war surgeon, advocated the consumption of wine the day after an operation on a wound. "However, the wine" he said, "must be the best that can be found; light, aromatic and agreeable to drink. One can give a 'chopine parisienne' [a small bottle of 50cl] with the morning meal and half a 'chopine' in the evening".

Arnaud de Villeneuse (1240–1320) had a special fondness for white wines: "giving less heat and less nourishment, they damage the brain less and provoke more urine than the others. They are more suitable for school children and students who must use wines that are conducive to understanding. Moreover, they are suitable for those who have a tired brain, either by nature or by accident."

Boccaccio on the other hand tells us that he held out against the plague by drinking wine with moderation.

The Renaissance

The Hippocratic principles as well as those of Galen, remained for a long time the standard by which all else was judged, since the pioneering work of Harvey and Pecquet on the circulation of blood and lymph in the body was recognised only very slowly.

The selection of medicines during the Renaissance was always dominated by plants. However, the dissemination of knowledge which characterised this period, helped considerably in making the medicinal properties of wine more widely known. One of the principal champions of wine during this period was none other than François Rabelais, though we tend to forget that he was a respectable doctor of the medical faculty at Montpellier. It was he who proclaimed loudly "the juice of the vine clears the mind and the understanding, chases sadness away and gives joy and understanding".

One of the things he particularly recommended for soothing a sting, was the flower of St John's Wort in hot wine. This was a time when medicinal recipes containing ground-up plants in wine were very popular: either for their antiseptic properties; for treating infections of the ear, nose and throat; soothing a cough; helping wet nurses lactate; combating jaundice, or for their aphrodisiac properties – to wit, the 41 remedies for "stoking-up the fire of love".

On the other hand, those suffering from gout were advised not to drink wine.

Michel de Montaigne, a contemporary of Rabelais was, in addition to being a man of letters and in particular a moralist (if not a philosopher), a wine grower from the Bordeaux region. He cured his kidney stones by drinking dry white wines and he never tired of letting everyone know how effective this treatment was. An indefatigable traveller always in search of culture and wisdom, he never missed the opportunity of staying on the shores of the lake of Geneva, so that he could undergo a cure at the small vineyard at Villeneuve, drinking the white wine known to have special diuretic properties. The philosophical wine lover declared his support for the principles of the School of Salerno in his essays, when he wrote: "I have heard Sylvius, the excellent doctor of Paris, say that to keep up the strengths of the stomach and not let them get heavy, it is good once a month to wake them up with a surfeit of wine and prick them so they do not become sluggish." These practices were also familiar to the Dutch humanist Erasmus, who had found the ideal remedy for his sluggish digestion in the wines of Beaune.

As far as Ambroise Paré is concerned, the surgeon of the Valois, he methodically used poultices of red wine to treat his patients wounded in combat on the field of honour. This form of treatment makes more sense when we are made aware of the antibiotic properties of many red wines – particularly those of the Médoc.

From the Age of the Enlightenment

As Molière has reminded us with humour, blood letting, purging and colonic irrigation (to use a modern term) were the triptych of all "serious" medication. But this does not mean that all reference to wine ceased during this period. Quite the contrary; wine continued to maintain its position as a mainline medicine. Thus Fagon, the personal physician to Louis XIV, the Sun King, would prescribe Champagne for his illustrious patient when he suffered from an attack of gout, to replace the Burgundy that he normally drank on a daily basis.

In the same way, the physician Helvetius, who was entrusted with the health of the Regent, prescribed wine as a medication for more than 20 out of 60 occasions. This famous doctor declared, in fact, that "we must not object to the moderate use of wine, as it useful if not necessary, to aid the digestion and strengthen the stomach of convalescents".

The chemist Fourcroy was also of this opinion when he wrote: "Wine is an excellent remedy for those who do not drink it regularly. It is a tonic, a stomatic, a corroborant [a giver of strength] and a very strong cordial."

At that time, the vast majority of members of the medical fraternity in France, as abroad, agreed to recognise medicinal properties in wine that went well beyond relieving digestive problems. It may be surprising, but this view is still generally held in Anglo-Saxon countries today.

It may be remembered that it was thanks to Cromwell on the pretext of returning to the "Reformation of Manners" that wine growing was suppressed in England where it was flourishing. From then on, the English became lovers of French wine – particularly Bordeaux. But even though they were forced to drink wine less frequently, they have never stopped treating themselves with it.

In the encyclopaedia of Diderot and d'Alembert, a long article is dedicated to the virtues of different wines: "The wines of Orléans strengthen the stomach...the wines of Burgundy are nourishing... The red wine of

Bordeaux is austere [bitter] and strengthens stomach tone, it troubles neither the head nor the operations of the mind, it improves with travelling and is perhaps the most health-giving wine in Europe. The wines of Champagne exhale a delicate smell that rejoices the brain."

Voltaire himself declared "a little wine taken with moderation is a remedy for the body and the soul".

In the nineteenth century

With the years and centuries that passed, the use of the medicinal aspects of wine became more refined and carried on developing. Thus Todd even managed to develop what he called "Ethylotherapy" – more commonly known as alcohol therapy.

Officially, wine was used to fight dysentery and cholera. In 1822, Magnesia, a French doctor, prescribed Claret specifically for this type of infection. In doing this, he merely prefigured what Rambuteau was to do in 1886, when he added wine to drinking water to combat a new epidemic of cholera. For there were many doctors like Chomel, Sabrazès and Mercadier, who noticed the bactericidal power of Médoc over the typhus and cholera bacillus.

In the same way, Gigon and Richet thought that Sancerre wines had a destructive action on coli bacilli – something that other doctors, such as the Viennese Pieck, had also noticed. It is interesting to note that this gentleman also recommended that polluted water should be cut with one third wine, in order to make it suitable for drinking.

For a long time, wine had been among the products used in enemas. However, it is in the nineteenth century that this practice was extended when it was realised that it was effective in treating anaemia dyspepsia, gastric ulcers, internal bleeding (particularly in childbirth), as well as tuberculosis.

But this period is also the great era of medicinal wines: 164 of them are listed in the Parisian pharmacopoeia of 1840. In 1893, 11% of the wine consumed by the Welfare Services in France was used to make medicinal wines – about 3.2 million litres in all. The essential worth of these medicines lay in the active ingredients of the plant extracts they

91

contained, using wine to maximise their effect. For example:

- Cinnamon wine, to stimulate hunger

- Gentian wine, to improve digestion

- Wormwood wine (using the leaf), to eliminate worms and as a digestive

- Wine and iron acetate, to fortify

- Opium wine and autumn crocus, against gout

- Quinine wine, to lower fever.

Among these, quinine wine and Mariani wine had considerable success, thanks to important publicity they received in the prestigious revues of the period, such as *Illustration*. And the famous surgeon of that time from Lyon, Professor Villard, actively supported this promotion by signing the slogan which maintained that "the bistoury [a small scalpel] begins the healing, Mariani wine completes it".

As far as "athletes' wine" was concerned, which combined coca and the cola nut, the idea was taken up by an American chemist who, because he had no wine available, decided then to replace wine with sugared water. We now all know of course what happened when a firm from Atlanta then added carbonic acid to the concoction....

At the end of the nineteenth century, there were even doctors who had no qualms in maintaining that the daily diet of bread could be replaced by wine. We know, for instance, that a certain Dr Jules Guyot said in 1866 that if a family of four wanted to remain strong and active, they "should drink at least 1,500 litres of wine per year, that is about 1 litre per person per day".

In a period when the struggle against alcohol began, Dr Guyot who was one of the main protagonists in the debate, made a distinction between "natural wine, that nourishes and is beneficial" and the depraved distilled alcohols like absinthe that were beginning to ravage society at that time. The good doctor expressed the wish in his campaign that the worker would abandon the tavern, a den of vice, to return to his family – the "sanctuary of wine".

In the same spirit, Frédéric Pasy declared in a congress: "Do you want to prevent people going down the road of alcohol addiction? If so, place wine, healthy natural wine, in their path to ensure that alcohol does not devour them in the end."

Advertising posters of this period proclaim that "Wine is Health", with the blessing of the medical faculty featuring on the backdrop.

Even the great Pasteur made his contribution to this promotion, in announcing without reserve that "wine is the healthiest and most hygienic of drinks"; though this did not prevent him from campaigning together with the anti-alcoholic leagues that were mainly concerned with the evils of distilled alcohol, and absinthe in particular. The horror with which this drink was seen by the French in the nineteenth century is hard to imagine: Emile Zola's *The Dram Shop* (1877) gives us some clue.

In the twentieth century

While the anti-alcohol lobby was making the world more aware of the evils of alcohol abuse, wine in the twentieth century has not ceased to have its advocates among the more eminent members of the medical profession.

In 1904, Dr Gauthier – a member of the Institute of the French Academy of Medicine – approved the responsible consumption of wine when he said: "It is a precious drink as long as a dose of 1 gram of alcohol per kilo is not exceeded each day." Which would amount to about a litre of wine for a person weighing 80 kilos – or just over 2 pints for someone weighing 12st. 8lbs.

Many medical papers praise the virtues of wine; Claret in particular, for its magnesium, lithium, zinc and iron content.

In 1930, Dr Cuvier and Professor Perrot (Professor of Medicine at the Faculty in Paris) drew the attention of the world yet again to the medicinal properties of wine. A year later, André Tardieu founded the National Committee of Propaganda for Wine, furnishing schools with literature which informed the pupils that " a litre of wine with 10° of alcohol, has the same nutritional value as 900g of milk, 370 g of bread or 5 eggs"!

In 1934, during the Second National Congress of the "Médecins Amis des Vins de France" – which sounds much more grand in French than it does in English! – Dr Eylaud proposed what almost amounted to a "Codex of wine therapy" based on the exclusive use of wines from the Bordeaux.

In this exhaustive list of therapeutic indications, it says that "all the wines of Bordeaux can be used employing the usual methods, which are:

1. *By mouth* – which is the most usual way.

2. *Via the rectum* – as an enema
   (recommended by Professor Aran, Professor Foussagrives and Dr. Houssay).

3. *By immersion* – in baths
   (recommended by Dr Simon and Professor Lereboullet)

4. *Intravenously* – diluted or undiluted (This involves no danger providing the volume does not exceed one-tenth of a cc for every kilo of body weight. This would correspond to an 8cc injection of wine for a person weighing 80 kilos.)"

In 1935, Dr. Dougnac appointed himself apostle of "wine therapy" as a way of overcoming alcoholism. Using numerical evidence, he shows that in wine growing regions there is less alcoholism (a fact that still holds true in 1997) and that people live longer in the region of Bordeaux than elsewhere in France.

In 1936, the firm of Nicolas (wine merchants) published a booklet entitled "My doctor: Wine", illustrated by the well-known artist Raoul Dufy, which was a collection of messages in favour of wine coming from leading medical figures.

After the Second World War, progress in scientific research has placed more and more "chemical" medicines in the hands of allopathic medicine, which have very quickly obscured the remedies and natural medication of the past. From now on it is the little pill that cures as soon as the illness manifests itself that is king. Gradually, the concept of preventative medicine that underlay the counsel of doctors to prescribe wine, falls more and more into disuse.

However, since 1975, when the last medicinal wines disappeared from the Codex of Pharmacopoeia, a certain number of scientists and doctors have continued to work semi-secretly on the therapeutic elements in wine. In the nineteenth century, men of science like Pasteur, who maintained wine was good for health, did so on the basis of experimentation, observation but also by intuition and therefore through personal conviction. The doctors who are now relaunching the question of the medicinal powers of wine do so on scientific bases that demonstrate their case clearly.

Thus Dr Maury (in 1978 with *Caring for Yourself with Wine* followed in 1988 by *Medicine through Wine*) then Dr Tran Ky (who has analysed the therapeutic virtues of Champagne, Claret and Burgundy wine in his *Modern Molecular Biology*) have been the precursors of the important work conducted in recent years by Professors Masquelier and Renaud, when they laid the foundations of the *French Paradox*.

CHAPTER 6

WINE, THE BEST PROTECTOR AGAINST HEART DISEASE

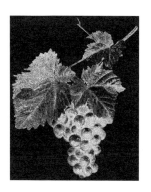

THE "FRENCH PARADOX"

While in many countries of the world, people still die of hunger or suffer from the effects of malnutrition, in the industrialised countries with their abundance of food, people are the victims of "civilisation sickness". As each day goes by, we become more aware that these grave health problems may be ascribed to perverse dietary patterns that have developed in western countries over the last half-century.

In developed countries, the main cause of death is linked to cardio-vascular diseases. In the United States, they are the cause of one-third of all deaths. These cardiovascular conditions are often associated to other illnesses, such as diabetes, obesity or arterial hypertension, and they are generally accompanied by atheroma or fatty deposits forming on the walls of the blood vessels. These fatty deposits, formed by LDL cholesterol (or "bad" cholesterol), cause constrictions in the blood vessels which then deteriorate, become more rigid and result in what is called atherosclerosis.

The blood, which also has a tendency to thicken, forms clots that can, in extreme cases, block an artery. According to where this obstruction occurs, different types of pathology can arise: myocardial infarction (heart attack) caused by blockage of the coronary arteries that supply the heart; an ischaemic cerebral accident (stroke) caused by blockage of the arteries that supply the brain; arteritis of the lower limbs or again a thrombosis of the artery supplying the retina.

For several decades, the United States has been particularly affected by deaths brought about by cardiovascular disease. In 1990, one and a half million Americans were victims of myocardial infarction and more than a third of these died as a result. Faced with this almost sacrificial slaughter of adults in the full flow of their lives at less than 60 years of age, this country, which prides itself on its vigour and its humanity, really had no option but to react.

With customary rigour, the Americans decided to analyse the mortality rates in other developed countries to see whether the conditions in those countries were any different from their own. The study conducted in 1980 on 7,000 people by Professor Ducimetière, revealed that there were great disparities between the various countries of the Western world. In particular, they showed that the incidence of heart attacks on the mortality rate was 36% to 56% lower in France than it was in the United States.

Even more surprising was the discovery that this difference was as pronounced when comparing people of the same age as it was when comparing against the same cardiovascular risk factors (blood pressure, blood cholesterol levels, consumption of saturated fats and smoking). In this way, the scientists came to realise that eating the same quantity of fat as the Americans, having the same or higher average cholesterol levels, the French had a much lower coronary mortality rate.

The "French Paradox" was born! Having tracked cholesterol and pursued fats in foodstuffs in an obsessive and almost paranoid way, now the American scientists were confronted by something that was quite incomprehensible.

In 1990, the statistics of the WHO (World Health Organisation) confirmed the following data:

Annual mortality rate per 100,000 men (corrected for age)

Country	Deaths due to Heart Disease	Average Cholesterol level	Fats consumed as a percentage
U S A	240	2.09 g/l	46
France	91	2.33 g/l	45

The major survey MONICA (MONItoring CArdiovascular Diseases) was launched in 1981 by WHO. Based on information collected from 40 centres in 20 countries, it gave a detailed picture of the situation in Europe.

Annual mortality rate per 100,000 men (corrected for age)

Cities	Country	Deaths due to Heart Disease	Total Deaths
Glasgow	United Kingdom	380	1179
Lille	France	105	1041
Strasbourg	France	102	887
Toulouse	France	78	575

From this we can see that the so-called "French Paradox" is the product of an oversimplification. It is perhaps better to talk of a North-South gradient. In fact, in the North of France, the number of deaths due to coronary heart disease approaches those of Anglo-Saxon countries. Only Toulouse in the South, can claim to be truly representative of the "paradox".

Thanks to the science of epidemiology, which studies the relationship between the risk factors and the illnesses where the correlations indicate preventative action, it is possible for us to interpret the data correctly. We are thus able to see that it is the diet which makes the difference. In fact, an analysis of the epidemiological data leads to four conclusions:

1. Death due to coronary heart disease is proportional to the consumption of saturated fats and fresh milk products. It will be noticed in the graphs – see Appendix 2 – that the Anglo-Saxon countries that eat the highest amount of saturated fats (of animal origin) – Chart 1 – and drink the most milk – Chart 2 – have a high level of mortality. This is not the case with Japan, which is a large consumer of fish (containing polyunsaturated fats), or Latin countries around the Mediterranean, which consume olive oil (monounsaturated fat) and little or no milk.

2. It is important to realise that the consumption of cheese containing saturated fats, has no bearing on the results. The reason for this is already known: the fats from the cheeses are not totally absorbed by the intestines for they combine with calcium to form "soaps" which are expelled in the faeces. This is the reason the French, who are big cheese eaters, figure so well in the chart – see Chart 3.

3. The mortality rate due to coronary heart disease is inversely proportional to the consumption of fruit, vegetables and vegetable fats (with the exception of palm oil) – see Chart 4.

4. The mortality rate due to coronary heart disease is inversely proportional to the consumption of alcohol. But among alcoholic drinks, it is wine that is the most effective in preventing cardio-vascular disease.

In other terms, the more wine drunk per head of the population, the lower the risk of dying from coronary disease. The data – see Chart 5 – shows very clearly that wine-drinking countries, such as France, Greece, Italy and Spain, are the ones where the death rates are lowest.

Conversely, Anglo-Saxon and Nordic countries have a risk factor that is three or even four times greater than France. Finland is a case in point. It is interesting to note that the curve plotted for wine is an exponential one, showing that the lower the consumption of wine, the greater the risk of death by coronary heart disease.

Thus, among the four factors studied (saturated fats, milk products, fruit and vegetables, and wine) there is irrefutable evidence that the determining factor in the "French Paradox" is the consumption of wine.

This is what was underlined in 1992, by Professor Renaud in an article in one of the most prestigious medical journals in the world, the *Lancet*. He had in fact broken the news of his findings through the American television programme *Sixty Minutes* on 17 November 1991. The effect of this programme on the United States was profound and since then, the amount of wine drunk there has gone up considerably.

However, preventing heart attacks by modifying your diet is at odds with drinking little or no wine. In fact, if we compare the dietary habits of the population of three French cities, we will see that there are significant variations in the consumption of other foods.

Comparative dietary habits in three French cities in grams per day as compiled by the MONICA survey

Food	Strasbourg	Toulouse	Lille
Bread	164	225	152
Vegetables	217	306	212
Fruits	149	238	160
Butter	22	13	20
Cheese	34	51	42
Vegetable Fats	16	20	15
Wine	286	383	267

(Source: after Jost and colleagues, 1990)

The Mediterranean regions of France have a natural preference for olive oil, fruit and vegetables, pulses (dried beans and lentils) and wine. In the more northerly regions of France, the preference is for butter, potatoes and beer. As we have seen earlier in the chapter, the mortality rate associated with cardiovascular disease is appreciably higher in cities like Lille and Strasbourg in Northeast France, than it is in the South of France at Toulouse.

Then again, if we examine the Mediterranean area a little more closely, taking the mortality rate in the United States as our reference, we find some striking differences.

Annual mortality rate per 100,000 inhabitants

Country	Deaths due to coronary disease	All deaths
U S A	424	961
Italy	200	1092
Crete	9	627

(Source: Seven Country Studies, Keys 1980)

From these figures it would appear that Crete is not only the country with the lowest level of deaths due to cardiovascular disease, it is also the country with the longest life expectancy. Perhaps, rather than talk about the "French Paradox", it might be more appropriate to talk about the "Cretan Paradox" or the "Mediterranean Paradox".

If we compare the dietary differences between the United States and Crete, we come up with the following data:

Eating habits – grams per person per day

Food	Crete	U S A
Bread	380	97
Pulses	30	1
Vegetables	191	171
Fruit	464	233
Meat	35	273
Fish	18	3
Added Fat	95	33
Alcohol/Wine	15	6

(Sources: Keys and Kronshout)

ALCOHOL AND HEALTH

There seem to be several factors that can be identified as helping to reduce the risks of cardiovascular disease like fruit, vegetables, fish and unsaturated fats. But the only "food" that has been shown to have a positive correlation, is wine. All the studies that have so far been conducted in the world agree on this point.

These studies show, in fact, that with a moderate consumption of wine – that is, from one to four glasses of wine a day – deaths due to heart attacks fall by 15% to 60% when compared to people who drink no wine at all. Beyond this level, the protective effect of wine tends to diminish.

This protection, which is expressed statistically as a J or a U curve, shows that 24 to 34 grams of alcohol in the form of wine (one 10 cl glass of 12° wine = 10 g of alcohol) is the amount which ensures the lowest incidence of coronary heart disease.

On the other hand, those that do not drink alcohol as well as those that drink too much (< 60 g of alcohol per day) have a higher risk of dying of coronary heart disease. In fact Professor Renaud has pointed out that those not drinking wine account for 76% of deaths due to coronary heart disease.

Deaths per 100,000 people, as a function of the number of glasses containing alcohol drunk per week

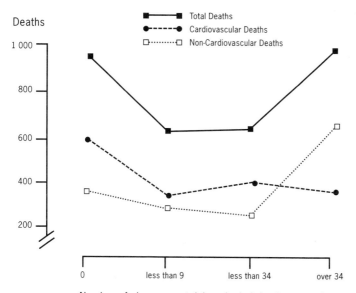

Number of glasses containing alcohol drunk per week

(Source: Marmot 1991)

This beneficial effect of alcohol (and more particularly wine) on the cardiovascular system, has been known for a long time. But most doctors, at least those in France, were afraid of being accused of promoting alcoholism.

And yet as early as 1951, an American cardiologist Professor White, observed that one of the best "heart remedies" after nitric derivatives (*trinitrin*), was alcohol. Likewise, in a study conducted in 1979, Dr Saint-Léger showed that when compared to a person drinking water, the risk of a wine drinker suffering a heart attack was 30% lower for a man and 39% lower for woman.

But it was in 1990 that the major study by Bofetta and Garfinkel showed accurately the variation in cardiovascular deaths and the total number of deaths due to the consumption of alcohol – see Appendix 2, Chart 6.

Bofetta Study 1990

Wine consumption	Total risk of death	Risk of death by heart attack
1 glass/day	0.84	0.79
2 glasses/day	0.93	0.80
3 glasses/day	1.02	0.83
4 glasses/day	1.08	0.74
5 glasses/day	1.22	0.85
6 glasses/day	1.38	0.92
Occasional drinker	0.88	0.86
Non drinker	1.00	1.00

This study of wine drinkers uses the person who does not drink wine as the basic reference, to whom an arbitrary Death Risk Index (DRI) of 1 is given. If a wine drinker has a DRI of 0.83, that means that his or her risk of death is 17% lower than the reference. On the other hand, an index of 1.36 would correspond to an increased risk of 36% with respect to the reference non-wine drinker.

In order to reduce the risk of dying from a heart attack without increasing the risk of dying from some other cause, the figures from this survey would suggest the optimum amount of wine to drink is two glasses a day. However, the lowest risk of dying from a heart attack occurs when you drink 4 glasses of wine a day: apparently it is a massive 26% lower than it would have been had you remained teetotal. Though it should be added, that if you do drink 4 glasses of wine a day, the chance you will die from something other than a heart attack is increased by 8%. If you drink 5 glasses of wine a day, the chances of dying from a heart attack are still lower by 15%, but the likelihood of dying from other causes is 22% higher. At this point, most people would conclude that the disadvantages of drinking wine outweigh the advantages.

The health advantages of drinking wine are much more pronounced if you do not smoke. Studies conducted in Framingham show that out of 100,000 smokers who did not drink alcohol, 28 died of coronary heart disease, as against 5.7 from a similar sample of non-smokers drinking between 3 and 7 glasses of wine a day.

In the case of women, the risk of cardiovascular disease is lower before the menopause. This appears to be due to the protection given by their hormonal system, because after the menopause the risk factor is identical to that for men.

An American study conducted in Boston by Fush on 65,700 women between the ages of 34 and 65, revealed the following risk factors:

Wine consumption	Risk factor
Non drinkers	1.00
1-2 glasses per day	0.83
3 glasses per day	0.88
4 glasses per day	1.19

Over three and a half glasses a day, wine ceases to protect women from cardioascular disease.

In addition to its beneficial effects on coronary disease, a study conducted on more than 22,000 medical doctors of both sexes in the United States (*Circulation* 1997, 95, 3, 577) showed that those having 1 or 2 alcoholic drinks a day had a 37% lower risk of developing arteritis in the legs than those having only one or less than one.

However, all those familiar with epidemiology know that a correlation does not constitute a formal proof of causality. As Professor Apfelbaum has pointed out "the fact that France has the largest number of Renault cars and the highest level of liver cirrhosis should not lead us to conclude that driving a Renault will increase the risk of becoming cirrhotic".

To affirm the causality of a correlation, it is necessary to undertake a study of secondary prevention. For example, you take a group of people who are ill (having had a heart attack, for example) and who have been advised to follow a precise diet. Subsequently you verify whether the advice given has effectively prevented the reccurrence of another severe attack.

It is this experience of secondary prevention which Professor Renaud has conducted on subjects who were at risk after having been the victims of a myocardial infarct (heart attack).

Two groups of patients were set up: one received "classical" dietary advice; the other a Mediterranean-type diet, incorporating wine.

The result of this study was quite spectacular, since Professor Renaud observed a reduction of 76% in the reccurrence of myocardial infarction in the second group as compared to the first group. No medicine known to us today has achieved such results.

It was thought for a long time that all alcoholic drinks had the same beneficial effects on the cardiovascular system. Until in 1981, Professor Renaud showed in a study that, compared to other alcoholic drinks, wine (particularly red wine) offered the best protection against atheroma experimentally induced in rabbits.

Alcoholic drink	Reduction in arterial atheroma
Beer	-10%
Whisky	-28%
White Wine	-30%
Red Wine	-70%

In 1990, Dr Saint-Léger had closely matching results in a similar series of experiments:

Alcoholic drink	Reduction in arterial atheroma
Whisky	-16%
White Wine	-23%
Red Wine	-63%

In 1992, Klatsky from California published the results of a study that he had conducted for seven years on 129,000 people. Here too it was shown that compared to other alcoholic drinks, wine gave 40% better protection against cardiovascular disease.

And finally, in 1995 one last study on 12,000 people was published by Gronboek. This was the so-called *Danish Study* (Appendix 1), and it set the seal on all the research that had preceded it.

Deaths from cardiovascular disease, based on a non-alcoholic drinker with a risk factor of 1

Alcohol consumption	Beer	Wine	Spirits
Never	1.00	1.00	1.00
Once a Month	0.79	0.69	0.95
Once a Day	0.87	0.53	1.08
1-2 glasses a day	0.79	0.47	1.16
3-5 glasses a day	0.72	0.44	1.35

Deaths from other causes, based on a non-alcoholic drinker with a risk factor of 1

Alcohol consumption	Beer	Wine	Spirits
Never	1.00	1.00	1.00
Once a Month	0.82	0.86	0.80
Once a Day	1.02	0.75	0.92
1-2 glasses a day	0.96	0.80	1.81
3-5 glasses a day	1.22	0.50	1.86

This study demonstrates quite clearly that wine is more effective than either beer or spirits in reducing the risk of cardiovascular disease. One of the interesting results of this study is that drinking more than two glasses of beer a day increases the risk of death from causes other than cardiovascular disease by 22%.

In the *Scandinavian Med. Soc. Journal* 1996, (24, 107–113), Messner studied the mortality levels in Sweden during the period 1973–1987, basing his survey on 19,300 men and 2,050 women between the ages of 15 and 17. During the period investigated, the total consumption of alcohol remained the same, except the consumption of spirits declined by 7%, beer declined by 15%, and the consumption of wine went up by 75%. This change in drinking habits produced some positive results: the risk of dying from coronary thrombosis dropped by 15% in the case of men and 28% in the case of women.

But in addition to the kind of alcoholic drink consumed, the way in which it is drunk is also important. Drinking alcohol during the course of a meal as is customary in France, is more beneficial for you than drinking it on an empty stomach as the Anglo-Saxons tend to do.

This said, it is of paramount importance to remember that the frequency of consumption is the essential factor in reducing the risk of cardiovascular disease: *wine taken in moderate quantities every day and, if possible, at every meal, is the way of ensuring the best protection.* Over indulgence at the weekend or at irregular intervals, which often happens to be the case in northern countries, is of no use at all – in fact, it can actually be harmful. A little later on, we shall come to the reasons for saying this, when we study the physiological action of wine in more detail.

Bearing in mind all these studies, it is important to recognise that moderate, regular consumption of alcohol helps reduce the risk of cardiovascular disease. But of those alcoholic drinks, it is wine – and particularly red wine – which gives the best guarantee of protection. To do so in the most effective way, the following three conditions must be fulfilled:

1. No more than four glasses of wine should be drunk each day

2. Wine should only be drunk during meals

3. Wine should be drunk regularly on a daily basis.

Obviously, this advice is intended only for those who enjoy good health, have not been alcoholics or do not run the risk of inheriting alcoholism, are not drug dependent and are not undergoing medical treatment which would preclude them from drinking alcohol.

Until now, there has been no official independent organisation that has officially supported this advice, which is based on hundreds of very serious studies conducted in most of the countries in the West.

The World Health Organisation is very embarrassed and rightly so. This organisation, an offshoot of the United Nations, has as one of its main tasks that of recommending, as objectively as possible, all health measures that will improve the health of everyone across the world. On several occasions, its representatives have explained that they have refused to make any statement in favour of even a moderate consumption of wine, for fear of being misrepresented. And so the WHO, like the *Académie de Médecine* in France, leaves it to the medical profession to spread the news.

On the other hand, it has been a real godsend for those in the wine trade to discover that they can use authentic scientific statements to bolster their business. This they have done in a serious and moderate way, for it is in their interest not to be accused of hyperbole.

111

HOW WINE HEALS

In addition to ethyl alcohol with its power to inhibit cardiovascular disease, there are a further 800 or so substances in wine, of which only a few have been studied in depth.

We shall review those few substances that have been studied to date and see what effect they have on our health – bearing in mind, of course, that further discoveries will be made before the list is finally completed sometime in the future.

First of all we will return to the protective properties of wine with regard to coronary disease, in order to have a better understanding how this comes about. Then we will examine the protective properties of wine with regard to other aspects of our health.

Cardiovascular protection

Ethyl alcohol is not the only element responsible for the positive effects of wine in cardiovascular disease protection: if that were the case, all alcoholic drinks would have the same properties.

There are in fact, other substances in wine, like polyphenols, glycerol, soluble fibres and aspirin, which make it into one of the finest medications against cardiovascular disease to be had.

Wine contains about 80 grams of alcohol per litre. If you consider that there are about eight 12.5 cl glasses in a litre, one glass of wine contains 10 grams of alcohol. The exact amount of alcohol in a litre will vary according to the alcohol rating of the wine in the bottle:

Wine rated at 9°, will contain 75 grams of alcohol per litre

Wine rated at 10°, will contain 80 grams of alcohol per litre

Wine rated at 11°, will contain 88 grams of alcohol per litre

Wine rated at 12°, will contain 96 grams of alcohol per litre.

The amount of alcohol in wine is dependent, as we know, on the amount of sugar present naturally in the grapes or added in chaptalisation.

On the physiological level, wine acts in two ways: on the blood and on the walls of the blood vessels. That is to say, it acts both on the conduit and the contents.

Effects of alcohol on lipids in the blood

Atheroma (changes on the walls of the arteries which can lead to heart attacks and thrombosis) are encouraged by various factors: a high level of LDL-cholesterol (bad cholesterol); a low level of HDL-cholesterol (good cholesterol): a high level of Lipoprotein a (Lpa); a high level of triglycerides and a high level of fibrinogen.

Effects of alcohol on LDL-cholesterol

When large amounts of alcohol are drunk, the amount of LDL-cholesterol increases dramatically. This is what happens to casual drinkers who suddenly drink a lot. As we know, this is a fairly frequent habit of Anglo-Saxons, particularly those in Northern Europe, who set out to get drunk at weekends or when they go out together.

On the other hand, it has been noticed that moderate but regular drinkers have a slight reduction in their level of LDL-cholesterol. Studies have revealed that in a group of men between 30 to 47 years of age, drinking a bottle (75cl) of wine each day lowered their LDL-cholesterol level from 1.41 to 1.19 g/l when compared to a period when they drank no wine at all.

Atheroma lesions due to the deposit of lipids on the walls of the arteries, are more likely to lead to a heart attack when the fats have oxidised. We already know about the antioxidant action of polyphenols in wine, which is particularly powerful. We know, for instance, that a concentration of only 10 micromoles per litre will inhibit oxidation by about 86% and a concentration of 20 micromoles per litre will inhibit oxidation completely. As the graph will show below, this antioxidant action is much stronger than vitamin E, which is often used as the benchmark.

Percentage of oxidised LDL

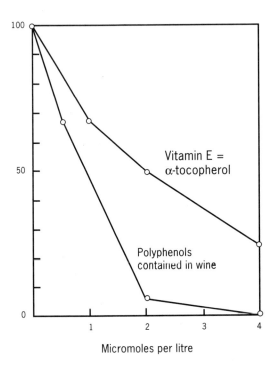

(Sources: FRANKEL E. N. Lancet, 1993, 341, 454–457)

Effects of alcohol on HDL-cholesterol

To understand the phenomenon properly, we should remind ourselves that HDL-cholesterol is made up of two subdivisions. HDL2 protects the cardiovascular system: it cleans the arteries of their fatty deposits. HDL3, on the other hand, has no particular protective role to play. It is understandable, therefore, that interest in increasing HDL-cholesterol depends on its quality, that is to say the amount of HDL2 that it contains.

For a long time, specialists in the field have given different advice regarding the effects of alcohol on each of the sub-divisions of HDL. Recent studies have shown greater uniformity of thought by clarifying the following points:

The effects of wine alcohol on HDL-cholesterol

Alcohol consumption grams per day	Corresponding number of glasses	Effects on HDL	Effectiveness
<40	1-3	Clear increase of HDL2 Marked increase of HDL3	Weak
60-80	6-8	Marked increase of HDL2 Weak increase of HDL3	Strong
<80	9+	No increase of HDL2 No increase of HDL3	None

(Source: Gaziano 1993)

From this table it would appear that 6 to 8 glasses of wine per day would create the best conditions for increasing the quantity of HDL-cholesterol, thanks to HDL2, and thereby increasing its protective power on the cardiovascular system.

With men aged between 30 to 47, HDL-cholesterol changes in the following manner as a result of wine having been consumed:

	Total HDL mg/l	HDL2 mg/l	HDL3 mg/l
No wine	43.5	5.7	37.7
75cl wine per day	49.4 (+14%)	10.4 (+82%)	39.0 (+3.4%)

(Source: Contaldo 1989)

It should be pointed out, meanwhile, that this beneficial increase in HDL-cholesterol will only occur if the liver is functioning normally and is not affected by cirrhosis or hepatitis. In addition, this increase works more effectively for the slim than for the fat, and for men rather than for women. But we should remind ourselves yet again that these beneficial effects can only be realised if wine is taken daily.

In other words, the beneficial effects will not occur for those that drink wine irregularly. We shall even see later on that drinking sporadically – say only at weekends – can be particularly dangerous.

115

The importance of daily consumption is clearly shown in a study conducted by Ridker in 1990.

Wine consumption	HDL-cholesterol (mg/l)
Rarely or never	44
Monthly	43
Weekly	46
Daily	50 (+13.5% compared to a non-drinker)

However, we should bear in mind that there are very big variations in the increase of HDL-cholesterol, depending on the individual: for the same amount of alcohol, it can vary from 14% to 72%.

This is explained by the influence other parameters can have on the level of HDL-cholesterol: the degree of hyperinsulinism, the percentage of body fat and its type, as well as the importance of physical activity or even heredity. There are in fact, people who respond well to alcohol and others who respond badly. Some recent studies conducted by Fumeron in 1995 would seem to indicate that this difference is genetic in origin [1].

It is generally believed that the action of alcohol on HDL and LDL-cholesterol only accounts for 50% of the protection given by wine against coronary heart disease.

The action of alcohol on Lipoprotein a

Lipoprotein a (Lpa) is an independent cause of atheroma and is therefore one of the factors associated with the risk of artherosclerosis.

---

1 The gene that codes the response of HDL-cholesterol to alcohol has two alleles; B1 and B2. Only individuals having the allele B2 would have this increase in HDL-cholesterol. This difference may be explained in the following manner: for lipids to be deposited in the arteries, a protein has to be present that transfers cholesterol onto lipoproteins of high density (HDL) or low density (LDL). People having the allele B2 will have a lower level of this protein CETP (Cholesterol Ester Transfer Protein) and thus a lower level of LDL-cholesterol and a higher level of HDL-cholesterol.

Encouraging studies have shown that drinking red wine helps to limit the levels of Lpa; white wine, on the other hand, has only had the effect of limiting the increase.

The action of alcohol on triglycerides

An excess of triglycerides has now been recognised as a real cardio-vascular risk factor, independent of cholesterol level.

Drinking too much alcohol can lead to a high level of triglycerides in the blood (over 15 g/l) And with people who are hypersensitive to alcohol, even a reasonable consumption of say 3 glasses of wine per day can be enough to keep the level critical.

Very often, eating too many sweet things or more generally carbo-hydrates with a high glycaemic index, like potatoes and foods made with refined flour, normally cause an abnormal level of triglycerides in the body. To control the problem, it is usually sufficient to reduce the intake of these foods or eliminate them entirely from the patient's diet.

Finally, non-insulin dependent diabetes mellitus (NIDDM), obesity and medication are sometimes all that is required to explain the excess of triglycerides – an excess that can be suppressed if the causes are brought under control.

The effects of alcohol on insulin

There are two contributory factors associated with the risk of cardio-vascular disease: too high a level of insulin (hyperinsulinism) or a disturbance in the way the body uses insulin (insulin resistance). It has been shown that weak doses of alcohol, such as one glass of wine, reduce the importance of hyperinsulinism and increase the sensitivity of the cells to insulin. As a result, the likelihood of a coronary heart attack is reduced.

The effects of alcohol on hormone activity

Owing to the reduced level of oestrogens circulating in the body, a woman after menopause has an increased risk of coronary vascular disease. Alcohol has the advantage of raising the level of oestrogens in the blood slightly, by stimulating their production in the adrenal gland.

117

The effects of alcohol on blood coagulation

Blood that is "too thick" because its viscosity has increased is more susceptible to the formation of a blood clot that can block an artery with a thrombosis. Alcohol has the advantage of making the blood "more fluid" using three different mechanisms:

- According to Professor Renaud, it reduces the aggregation of blood platelets, which could lead to the formation of a clot in an artery narrowed by the formation of a plaque.

Consumption of alcohol – grams per day	Equivalent amount of wine – glasses per day	Level of platelet aggregation
1 – 5	½	0.74
5 – 0	½ – 3	0.56
+30	+3	0.35

From this table we can see that by drinking more than three glasses of wine per day in place of water, the platelet aggregation level is reduced by 65%. Epidemiological studies show that the level of platelet aggregation among the people in the Var region of the South of France is 55% lower (better, in other words) than the level recorded for the Scots. The fall in this aggregation is more pronounced among heavy fat eaters, particularly those eating saturated fats.

If you want to reduce the deposit of dangerous lipids or fats on your artery walls during the period immediately following a meal, drinking wine during the course of a meal rich in saturated fats is therefore not only a pleasure but an obligation. Conversely, having a sugared drink following a fat-rich meal, such as a hamburger, can only aggravate the likelihood of fats settling on the walls of your arteries. Without doubt, here we have another reason explaining the phenomenon of the "French Paradox".

- The second mechanism that causes alcohol to make blood more fluid is its action on fibrinogen. This is a substance that is also involved in the formation of blood clots. The effect may appear modest, but reducing fibrinogen by 1% leads to a 4% reduction in the risk of a coronary heart attack.

- And finally, the "fluidity" of blood is improved by the formation of a substance that helps to dissolve a clot: plasminogenic tissue activator (PTA). Wine increases the amount of PTA produced by the body.

Consumption of wine	Level of PTA – nanograms/ml
Rarely or never	8.12
1 – 3 glasses per month	9.06
1 – 6 glasses per week	9.69
2 glasses a day or more	10.89

It is interesting to note that wine continues to have this anticoagulant effect even when it is drunk on an empty stomach, providing it is consumed on a daily basis.

It is also the case that heavy bouts of drinking at the weekend can lead to a rapid drop in the binding property of the platelets. This in turn, can lead to haemorrhages or bleeding.

However, the gravest problem can occur in the day or days that follow a heavy bout of drinking. Passing abruptly from a period of overindulgence to a period of total abstinence, is liable to produce a "rebound effect" leading to sudden hypercoagulation of the blood and thrombosis.

Because of this mechanism, it must be stressed that wine should be drunk more-or-less on a regular basis and certainly not sporadically. Sporadic drinking at festivities or heavy cyclical drinking at weekends. as is the habit in Scandinavian countries, is extremely dangerous. On Monday, the battered partygoer will probably just drink water or milk if he is Anglo-Saxon, and will increase the risk of provoking a heart attack. In fact, cardiovascular accidents are very high and statistics show, moreover, that there is a greater concentration of heart attacks at the beginning of the week.

This should be enough to put Frenchmen on their guard. For in order to be at peace with their conscience, they have adopted the habit of drinking water at all week time meals and then proceed to make up for

119

lost time on outings and at the weekends. These days when travelling in France during the week, it is very sad to see business meals lubricated just with mineral water. These same abstemious managers then go on a binge at weekends, drinking wines and spirits as if their sole aim in life were to end up in an ambulance on Monday morning.

The effects of alcohol on blood vessels

Alcohol increases the diameter of the coronary arteries, allowing more blood to reach the heart and reducing the risk of cardiac ischaemia (failure of the blood supply to the heart).

Alcohol blocks the constrictions of the blood vessels, particularly vascular spasms due to stress. But there again, it is all a question of quantities, because too high a consumption of alcohol (above 60 grams, or six glasses of wine, a day) creates free radicals that oxidise LDL – and oxidised LDL lipids are very atherogenic.

Here is another reason for drinking wine daily but in moderate amounts. Only in this way is it possible to avoid the formation of free radicals and benefit from the antioxidant effect of polyphenols.

Polyphenols

These are antioxidant substances that are found mainly in wine. Their classification is fairly complicated because it has often changed. Researchers have not always been in agreement regarding the exact terminology to adopt. Without getting too technical, it is sufficient to say that there are several types of polyphenols: flavonoids, anthocyans (including tannins), flavonols (from which we get procyanidols and catechins), resveratrols, phenolic acids, coumarins and quinones.

Polyphenols are already present in the grape (as a percentage of the total amount found in the grape, 60% occur in the pips and more than 20% in the skin).

The cardiovascular protective mechanisms of polyphenols

Protection of the capillaries

Polyphenols contained in wine double capillary resistance and reduce the risk of haemorrhaging by a similar amount. Besides, there is a medicine (Endothelon) with a polyphenol base which aims to prevent haemorrhages by increasing the capillary resistance of the blood vessels.

Protection of collagen

It has been noticed that an atheroma is formed more easily when the proteins of the vascular walls have already deteriorated. The structure of these proteins is ensured by the collagen fibres that give the structure solidity and elasticity. The work done by Professor Masquelier has demonstrated that the polyphenols in wine (red wine in particular) reinforce the structure and solidity of collagen, thus preventing the formation of atheroma.

The powerful antioxidant effect of polyphenols

The aim of antioxidants is to trap free radicals. In the body, electrons are organised in pairs, with one exception: oxygen. Oxygen is in fact, the only molecule that has "celibate" or individual electrons. These are what are known as free radicals. However, like all celibates, free radicals have only one idea: to mate. They therefore go out and try to couple with some chromosome DNA and lipids associated with cellular membranes. As a result, the cell walls are altered: they become rigid and oxidise. The oxidation can be compared to the formation of rust on metal. It is in this way that oxygen, whilst absolutely indispensable for life, can become toxic.

Free radicals are created in large numbers by tobacco addiction, ultraviolet light, pollution, excessive physical activity, as with high-intensity sport, and alcohol excess. By their destructive action on cells, they contribute to the deterioration of the cardiovascular system, leading to the appearance of arterial hypertension and arteriosclerosis. In addition, they accelerate the ageing process in cells, particularly those in the brain.

121

Fortunately, our bodies have a defensive strike force – a battalion of antioxidising enzymes. But with age, the ranks of these battalions diminish and there are fewer and fewer antioxidising enzymes ready for the fray. Food must therefore come to our aid, supplying us with anti-oxidants like polyphenols, betacarotene, vitamins C and E, selenium and zinc.

Wine is important for two reasons. Firstly, a moderate consumption does not lead to the creation of free radicals. Most importantly, as the work of Professor Masquelier has shown, polyphenols in wine have a powerful effect against free radicals. It is important to underline that this antioxidising action of polyphenols in wine is particularly strong, because it is 50 times more effective than vitamin E, which is usually cited as the reference.

The positive effect of polyphenols on platelets

Several studies (Folts, Renaud, Bertelli 1995) have shown that as with alcohol, polyphenols inhibit the aggregation of platelets by limiting, however slightly, the rebound effect that comes with sudden abstention from alcohol, which was denounced earlier.

Polyphenol concentration in wines

The concentration of polyphenols in wine depends on the grape variety and the way the wine was made – for instance, the type of grape will influence time allowed for the must to stand. This is particularly the case with red wines. There are large concentrations of polyphenols in the skin of the black grape and extended contact between the grape juice and the skins during fermentation is therefore essential to ensure that as many of them as possible are released into the wine.

Polyphenol (resveratrol) concentrations in different types of red wine

Region	Concentration
Burgundy	7 mg/l
Oregon (USA)	6.2 mg/l
Bordeaux	6 mg/l
Beaujolais	3.5 mg/l
Australia	3.2 mg/l
South Africa	3 mg/l
Italy	2.2 mg/l
South America	2 mg/l

(Source: Karumanchiri, quoted by Jones p.113)

Red wines contain on average about 2,500 mg/l of polyphenols. White wines contain a tenth of this amount. However, in 1995 Professor Vinson showed that with the same concentrations, the polyphenols in white wines were more powerful than those in red wines.

Grape juice contains a fair concentration of polyphenols, but their antioxidant effect is less effective than those in wine. This is because alcohol is necessary for the proper absorption of polyphenols through the intestinal wall.

The recommended daily intake of polyphenols is set at 300 to 400 mg. This much is contained in two glasses of red wine. But let us remember that there are polyphenols – though perhaps not many – in foods other than wine: foods like fruit, vegetables, cocoa, olive oil and green tea. On the other hand, beer and cider that originally have polyphenols, have had most of them removed during the manufacturing process, in order to stabilize the product.

Glycerol

This is a sugar-alcohol that comes from the family of carbohydrates. In wine its average concentration is 80 g/l. Glycerol has the effect of reducing hyperinsulinism and insulin resistance. It also reduces lesions in the muscles associated with the arteries, which could allow atheroma to develop. In addition, it encourages dilation of the arteries which in turn reduces the risk of thrombosis. However, these effects are only apparent with strong doses, which would not occur just by drinking wine.

Fibres

Wine contains soluble fibres: pectins and gums. Their level will vary according to the type of vine stock. There are not many, for example, in Syrah or Chenin. However, there are lots in Alicante-Boucher – about 600 to 1,000 milligrams per litre. They give wine its soft character.

Apart from enhancing the action of polyphenols in the blood, soluble fibres reduce the absorption of fats – particularly saturated fats – through the intestines. They also reduce hyperinsulinism and insulin resitance, as we know, two important factors associated with atherosclerosis.

Aspirin

Aspirin has been used for many years by cardiologists for secondary prevention. Until now it has been one of the most effective medicines for reducing by 21% the recurrence of thrombosis or myocardial infarction after a bypass operation.

Aspirin acts by inhibiting platelet aggregation and by protecting against vasoconstriction, which reduces the passage of blood through the arteries still further. The normal dose prescribed is 160 milligrams per day. However, it does expose the patient to haemorrhages, gastro-duodenal ulcers and gastritis.

Several studies have shown that wine contains aspirin: about 30 milligrams per litre in white wines and rather more in red wine. It must be realised therefore that this anti-aggregating action combined with that of polyphenols and alcohol, gives wine – providing it is taken in moderation – medicinal properties as effective as aspirin, with far fewer risks of possible dangerous side effects.

It should be remembered that aspirin raises the level of alcohol in the blood. Taking an aspirin after drinking his two glasses of wine, a driver risks going over the limit of 50 milligrams of alcohol per litre of blood, which is currently the legal limit in France. Therefore, the moral of the story is that if you intend to drive a car, never take aspirin after you have drunk even very moderate quantities of alcohol.

In the light of all these studies demonstrating the beneficial effects of wine on the cardiovascular system based on a reasonable consumption of between two to four glasses of wine a day, it is quite evident that the therapeutic properties of wine are considerable. If you then consider that wine is effective not only at this primary level but also in preventing dangerous side effects at a secondary level, then wine is an ideal medicine that many modern medicines would be very happy to emulate.

CHAPTER 7

OTHER BENEFICIAL EFFECTS OF WINE

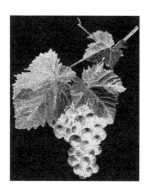

Much important scientific work carried out in many countries over recent years, has focused mainly on the cardiovascular protection afforded by wine. This has happened because cardiovascular disease is known to be a major cause of death and because various epidemiological studies have shown that the proportion of people liable to suffer coronary heart attacks is four times lower in countries where wine is drunk regularly.

Even if medical and health authorities are still coyly reluctant to make this information public, the news that wine drunk in moderation is good for health, is becoming more and more widely known thanks to the efforts of the media. Gradually wine has begun to emerge from the ghetto where it has been imprisoned for decades by the anti-alcohol lobby.

However, talk about the therapeutic qualities of wine is still largely limited to its dramatic effects on the cardiovascular system, though man has been well aware of its wider medicinal application for thousands of years. Both Hippocrates and Pasteur, separated by 2,000 years of history, have praised the healing effects of wine and scientific research in recent decades has repeatedly confirmed that what the ancients believed about wine was more than justified.

Wine fights infection

Professor Masquelier has shown very clearly that wine fights infection.

Antibacterial action of wine

If 10 million E coli bacilli are introduced into 50 cl of red wine, within half and hour they will all be dead. This powerful bactericide is not due to the acid (pH) or the alcohol present in wine, as might have been thought, but rather the anthocyanines (the blue colouring matter in plants) and cinnamonic acid.

Knowing its different components, it is possible to conclude that the bactericidal action of wine is quite extensive, including both germs (-) (Salmonella, Shigella, Colibacilli, Proteus) and germs (+) (Staphylococci, Streptococci, Pneumococci).

A recent study by Professor Weisse (BMJ 1995) has measured the anti-bacterial effect of wine as compared to alcohol and other antibacterial products like bismuth. His conclusions reinforce those of Professor Masquelier (Bulletin of the OIV, 1992).

The team of Professor Weisse has compared the effects of red and white wine as a bacterial agent on different strains of bacteria (Escherichia, Salmonella enteriditis and Shigella sonnei), against the effects of a bismuth solution, an alcohol solution and distilled water.

The results show that red and white wine act more quickly as an antibacterial agent on the bacteria strains studied, than does bismuth. As far as the alcohol solution is concerned, it has a no greater antibacterial effect than distilled water. Moreover, this study showed that given the same concentration of phenols, white wine reduces the number of bacterial colonies faster than red wine and bismuth was found to be less effective than either.

This study is interesting because it shows us clearly that the antibacterial effect observed with wine is not due to the alcohol content but to the polyphenol compounds that are released during fermentation.

As a result, we can understand better the rationale behind some of the ancient practices that have been handed down to us over the centuries. These, like drinking white wine with shellfish, particularly oysters, are firmly embedded in gastronomic tradition. Quite clearly, it is the best way of avoiding possible intestinal infection.

However, this bactericidal action of wine must be seen as essentially preventative. It would obviously be very unwise to treat a severe infection relying solely on the curative properties of red wine.

On the other hand, it has been shown that even a small quantity of wine introduced into polluted water in a tropical endemic zone can have an interesting prophylactic effect. Mixing together equal amounts of red wine and polluted water will make the water safe to drink.

In addition, when combined with naturally occurring vitamin C, the significant quantities of iron contained in wines like those from the Médoc can help the immune system to fight more effectively against infections.

Antiviral action of wine

Plants do not have an immune system, but they do have defence mechanisms to protect them against viral infections, as in the case of the vine. Experiments conducted in laboratories have shown that even diluted red wine will destroy the poliomyelitis virus and similar effects can be obtained using concentrations of a few milligrams of tannins or procyanide oligomeres. Identical results have been obtained with other viruses, like Coxakie and Herpes.

Studies have shown that this action is brought about by tannins locking onto and blocking the viral protein necessary for the virus to penetrate and infect the cell. This antiviral action of wine has been confirmed in man: wine drinkers who do not smoke are less likely to contract influenza than non-smokers who do not drink wine. Wine therefore has a preventative effect with regard to influenza infection.

Medical statistics at the workplace show that people who drink wine in moderation suffer less absenteeism as a result of infectious diseases than those who abstain.

Anticaries action of wine

It is known that caries is an infectious disease. During the process of transforming sugars in the mouth, *Streptococcus mutans* encourages the appearance of dental plaque, which later gives rise to the formation of caries. However, when the procyanides in wine lock onto the bacteria, they disrupt their action and prevent the formation of dental plaque.

The antiallergic action of wine

We know that certain polyphenols inhibit the enzyme histidine decarboxylase that transforms histidine (an inoffensive amino acid) into histamine, which is responsible for allergic reactions.

Finnish researchers have recently confirmed these experimental findings by showing that wine can limit difficulties associated with hayfever. Unfortunately, there are wines which are rich in histamines and can bring about allergic reactions in people who are hypersensitive. In the same way, a wine excessively strong in sulphites can bring about an asthma attack. In this latter case, it is advisable to select organic wines that contain few or no sulphites.

Wine is the best digestive

This is certainly one of the qualities which has been most recognised and appreciated in wine during the course of its history. Today, science gives us the explanation.

Action on the stomach

Wine protects against gastroduodenal ulcers by inhibiting the formation of histamine.

The studies of Peterson in 1986, showed that wine stimulates gastric secretions in the stomach, making it an effective aperitif. The author deduced that the amines in the wine (tyramine, dimethylamine, ethanolamine) give it this property. It is therefore reasonable to conclude that wine taken before a meal, will stimulate the secretion of digestive juices and particularly those that are responsible for the digestion of proteins.

Another study published in 1991 by Chacin, shows that alcohol on its own – say wine – has no beneficial effect on the mucous membrane of the stomach and that when its concentration is high (above 20%), its effect will be negative as it will inhibit gastric secretion.

This confirms that spirits (gin, whisky, vodka) taken before a meal as is sometimes customary, have absolutely no aperitif function and may even upset the digestion of foods eaten afterwards.

Action on the gall bladder

Certain components of wine like cinnamine acid, stimulate secretions from the gall bladder and, as a result, wine can make a considerable contribution to the digestion of a "heavy" meal by helping to accelerate the digestion of fats in the small intestine.

Action on the pancreas

It has been shown by Gin and Christiansen in 1992, that small doses of wine (1 or 2 glasses per meal) improves sensitivity to insulin, the pancreatic hormone entrusted with controlling sugar levels in the blood (glycaemia).

In adult Type II Diabetes or fat diabetes (so called because it goes hand-in-hand with excess weight), the pancreas has a tendency to secrete too much insulin (hyperinsulinism). However, this insulin is not recognised by the body and has little effect, giving rise to a condition called *insulin resistance.*

The pancreas then tries to lower the sugar level in the blood by secreting even more insulin, which in turn aggravates hyperinsulinism. It has been noted that small doses of wine taken daily, break this vicious circle of hyperinsulinism leading to insulin resistance, by improving the sensitivity of tissue to insulin and thereby contributing to an improvement in the diabetes.

Action on the small intestine

Wine causes a slight slowing down in the movements of the intestine. This lengthens the digestion time and allows the digestive enzymes to act more effectively.

Action on the large intestine

Wine has a very clear antispasmodic and antidiarrhoeic effect. It has been shown that this action is due to flavonoids and catechins. As far as bacterial diarrhoea is concerned and for want of a better way of putting it, wine is able to reduce the loss of liquids in the intestines by sterilising the infected area.

Wine and excess weight

A small quantity of wine (1 glass at the end of a meal) can lead to weight loss.

Wine contributes to reducing glycaemia and correcting the hyper-insulinism responsible for increasing weight. The lowering of insulin brings about reduction in weight by promoting the action of triglyceride lipase, responsible for breaking down fat reserves. It has been shown elsewhere (Bravo 1994) that catechin in wine increases the elimination of fat through the alimentary tract.

Anti-ionising action of wine

The antioxidising properties of wine have been used to reduce the formation of free radicals created by radioactivity – as happened in the wake of the Chernobyl nuclear disaster, when local medical teams found themselves unable to administer more conventional forms of treatment.

Wine delays ageing

Free radicals result from the oxidising process, which disturbs the structure of DNA in chromosomes as well as the structure of body cells. This process interferes with cell reproduction, for the cells no longer perform as well as those from which they originate.

To understand how these successive reproductions can bring about a progressive change in the cells, one need only to look at a photo-copying machine. If you photocopy a text many times using not the original but the last copy, the quality of the reproduced text becomes progressively less and less legible. Something similar occurs with the cells damaged by the free radicals, for each time they reproduce their quality deteriorates. In this way it is possible to understand the phenomenon of ageing in cells.

The best way of reducing these changes and preventing the phenomenon of ageing is to fight against the free radicals. Thanks to its abundance of polyphenols, the antioxidising effect of wine can be seen as an excellent means of combating the ravages of time.

However, the antioxidising action of wine is only effective in moderate quantities (2 glasses per meal), since too much alcohol is itself a generator of free radicals.

In 1933, Dr Dougnac demonstrated that longevity was more evident in wine growing regions.

Age Groups	The increase in life expectancy in the Médoc region as opposed to the whole of France, expressed as a percentage
60 – 64	+25%
65 – 69	+27%
70 – 79	+29%
80+	+46%

Dr Dougnac also made a comparison between the longevity of the inhabitants of the Calvados region where cider and strong spirits are drunk, and the inhabitants of the Gironde, who drink mainly Claret the wine of Bordeaux. This comparison is also very instructive:

Age Groups	The increase in life expectancy in the Gironde as opposed to the region of Calvados, expressed as a percentage
60 – 69	+35%
70 – 79	+33%
80 +	+65%

A more recent study in 1986 made by Dr Baspeyras has shown that the differences remain more or less the same today.

Perhaps we should not be surprised at this, since in France popular wisdom has always counselled the elderly to drink a glass of wine with each meal in order to enjoy a long and healthy life. And for my part, my grandmother who came from Bordeaux, followed this advice methodically and lived to the ripe old age of 102.

Science tells us today that red wine, rich in polyphenols, helps us live longer. Jeanne Calment, who only died this year having lived to the age of 122, always underlined the fact that she owed her exceptionally long life not only to the climate and cooking of her native Provence, but also to the port and chocolate that she had prescribed for herself on a daily basis – two foodstuffs particularly rich in polyphenols.

Besides this, let us remember that the tannins in wine (particularly red wine) are effective in preventing cataracts – a particular affliction of the elderly – by inhibiting the enzyme aldolase reductase which is indirectly responsible for this condition.

In addition, Professor Orgogozo (Paquid Study 1997) has shown that those who drink between ¼ and ½ litre of wine per day, have a 65% lower risk of developing Alzheimer's disease than those who drink no wine at all.

Sceptics have pointed out that Professor Orgogozo comes from the Bordeaux region and is therefore biased in favour of wine. And the same has been said of Professor Masquelier, who has been demonstrating since the early 1980s – sadly with little recognition – how wine can be effective in helping to control cardiovascular disease.

The anti-inflammatory action of wine

A few preliminary studies have shown that the polyphenols in wine (yet again!) could have an indirect anti-inflammatory effect by inhibiting the enzymes that trigger the phenomena of inflammation. However, little work has been done in this field, though in Japan and China, the anti-inflammatory polyphenol resveratrol is already being used clinically.

Wine improves iron absorption

The absorption by the body of iron contained in food, is increased when wine is drunk – particularly white wine. However, absorption is always improved when wine is taken during the course of the meal.

The anticancerous action of wine

It has been shown that wine drunk in reasonable amounts, can protect and lower the risk of getting cancer. It is known that free radicals are heavily implicated in the generation of cancer and we know that they can be inhibited by polyphenols.

Fibre also has an anticancerous action, proven at least for cancers of the rectum and large intestine. It has been shown too that aspirin helps prevent cancers developing in the oesophagus and the large intestine. We now know, of course, that polyphenols and aspirin are present in wine in significant quantities, together with some soluble fibre.

In 1996, Professor Clifford, from the University of California in Davis, conducted an interesting study on laboratory animals that developed spontaneous cancerous tumours. Compared with the control group fed on a standard diet, 80% of the animals fed on a diet containing a solid extract of wine (containing no alcohol) survived beyond the 80 days in which theoretically they should have died of cancer.

The authors stress therefore that high concentrations of polyphenol compounds in the blood resulting from a moderate consumption of wine, could well contribute to a delay in the appearance of cancerous tumours.

Whilst researching anticancerous molecules in no less than 600 plants, the team of Professor Pezzuto at Illinois University has shown the beneficial effects of the polyphenol resveratrol found in a Peruvian vegetable. It should be remembered that resveratrol[1] is present in large quantities in the skin of grapes and in red, rosé and white wines.

Wine is the best remedy for stress

In 1994, a study conducted by Lipton showed that if the effect of alcoholic drinks on the management of stress and the prevention of depression was analysed and transposed to a graph, a 'U' type curve emerged. That is to say that those who drink water or very little alcohol are as sensitive to stress as those who drink large amounts of alcohol. Only moderate drinkers of alcohol are able to manage stress relatively well and are less subject to depression.

1 Resveratrol is active in three stages of cancer:

   a) During the first stage at the beginning of the tumour, it acts as an antioxidant and blocks the cellular mutation of DNA

   b) In the second stage when the cancerous cells spread, it reinforces the immune system and inhibits the enzyme cyclo-oxygenase which causes the cancerous cells to grow and multiply

   c) In the third stage of development of the tumour, resveratrol slows down the spread of cancerous cells.

The study of resveratrol in mice demonstrated its effectiveness in inhibiting the development of skin cancer that had been induced chemically. In future publications, we look forward to confirmation that resveratrol is equally successful in man.

A preliminary study in this field was published in the United States in January 1997 in *The archives of internal medicine*: here it said that among people who take 2 to 6 glasses of alcoholic drink a week, the risk of dying from cancer is lowered by 21-28% when compared to those who take only 1 glass or less a week.

Sources: Science 10.01.97 – Circulation 1997 – 95, 3, 577.

In 1979, a survey in France asked a sample of people why they drank alcohol. The replies were as follows: beer was drunk to quench thirst (particularly when the weather was hot); aperitifs and digestifs were drunk "to join in with everyone else"; wine was drunk "to accompany meals" (79%).

It is interesting to note that nobody dared say that they also drank wine because it stimulates or tranquillises – in other words, for its anti-stress qualities – for fear of being misunderstood. This is understandable. Even if you dare talk with abandon about the hedonistic pleasures associated with drinking wine when showing your collection of wines to your friends, you may have considerably more difficulty in declaring publicly that you also drink wine to cheer yourself up or combat stress.

However, we should recognise that wine is really a stimulant. It combats anxiety and depression. It is even a hypnotic sedative. But are these really shameful effects we should not mention, because they offend current mores – because some people have always had a tendency to confuse wine with drugs, seeing any conviviality involving wine as the antechamber of alcoholism?

Which doctor today would dare recommend, even if he had prescribed it for himself, the moderate consumption of wine to shed inhibitions, increase self-confidence, temper anxiety or simply look at life through rose-tinted spectacles? But if wine is this "social elixir" which improves human relationships, can it be a crime or even just improper to use it? Providing we remember of course, that it can impair our performance when driving a car and therefore drink it with discretion.

We have seen that the consumption of wine in France has decreased dramatically. Perhaps this is the explanation (or at least one of the explanations) for the Frenchman's increasingly gloomy outlook on life these days.

French doctors should perhaps bear this in mind before they prescribe without question and to the considerable benefit of the pharmaceutical industry:

85 million boxes of tranquillisers

22 million boxes of neuroleptics

43 million boxes of antidepressants

67 million boxes of sleeping tablets.

Apart from the immense cost to the health service, they have made the French into the largest consumers of psychotropic drugs in the world. And I ask myself whether a good glass of wine might not be a more judicious prescription rather than a capsule of chemicals guaranteed to leave the patient with nothing but a host of unwanted side effects.

The benefits of wine for the cerebrovascular system

Cerebrovascular accidents (strokes) are due either to a haemorrhage or to an obstruction caused by arteriosclerosis and thrombosis of an artery supplying blood to the brain. In this latter case, the area of the brain that is deprived of blood will cease to function either temporarily or permanently. This can lead to paralysis, hemiphlagias (paralysis down one side of the body) and speech problems. If we leave on one side the absence of vascular spasm, the mechanism of the lesions suffered is fairly similar to what can happen in the case of the heart.

If wine, as has been widely shown, effectively prevents coronary atheroma, it follows that it can also prevent cerebral atheroma with the same effectiveness.

Several studies have in fact shown this to be the case, among which:

The Stampfer study in 1988

Wine in grams of alcohol/day	0	<15	15 to 50	60 to 140
Level of risk	1	0.7	0.4	0.8

The Plomäki study in 1993

Wine in glasses/day	0	2	5
Level of risk	1	0.5	1

In 1990, the Klosky study showed as well that two or three glasses of wine each day will help to prevent cerebral ischaemia – a lack of blood to the brain.

After the publication of *The French Paradox* proving the beneficial effects of wine in combating cardiovascular disease, several doctors challenged its findings, claiming that what had been accredited to wine in general could be accredited to alcohol in particular. They therefore pronounced that any alcohol, whether it be whisky, gin or beer could produce the same beneficial effects, so long as they were consumed regularly in moderate quantities.

However, we have seen in the preceding chapter that even if other alcohols can have beneficial effects on the cardiovascular system, it is wine that is by far the most effective. However, above all in this chapter we have seen that wine harbours an impressive array of therapeutic powers. Powers that make it a medicine in its own right.

CHAPTER 8

The Dangers of Excessive Consumption

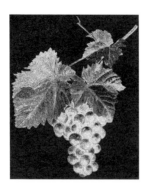

We have seen in previous chapters that wine is a food: consumed in moderation, it is not only nutritious it is also exceptionally healthy.

The key word though, is "moderation". As Hippocrates said: "it is the dose that makes the poison". This chapter has been written to stress this point with regard to wine.

Yet it should be noted that the threshold beyond which wine can have a negative effect is not the same for everyone. In general, women have a lower tolerance than men and there are variations in sensitivity within both the sexes.

The metabolism of alcohol

It is in fact the alcohol that introduces the risk factor. Once the wine is absorbed, the alcohol (ethanol) is metabolised by the action of the enzyme ADH (alcohol-dehydrogenase) into acetaldehyde. Through the action of a second enzyme ALDH (acetaldehyde-dehydrogenase), the acetaldehyde is transformed into acetate. The larger part of this acetate (about 70%) is expelled as heat. The rest is transformed into fats, notably triglycerides.

The enzyme ADH responsible for the metabolizing of alcohol operates in two organs: the stomach and the liver.

If the wine is consumed on an empty stomach, the enzyme ADH will have no time to act before the alcohol passes through the stomach into the small intestine, where it will be absorbed into the blood stream and taken to the liver. It is here that the ADH in the liver will begin to act on the alcohol, coping with about 100 mg of alcohol per kilo per hour.

That is to say:

- 6 gm alcohol per hour in a person weighing 60 kilos
- 7 gm alcohol per hour in a person weighing 70 kilos
- 9 gm alcohol per hour in a person weighing 90 kilos.

As soon as these amounts are exceeded, despite the intervention of another enzyme P450, alcohol passes into the blood circulation and

143

depending on the sensitivity of the individual, will manifest itself in a feeling of dizziness.

This is what can happen when we drink on an empty stomach and the alcohol gets into the bloodstream in less than twenty minutes.

When wine is drunk during a meal, the passage of alcohol is more gradual. It is generally accepted that in this case, the level of alcohol in the blood circulation reaches its peak about an hour after the last glass of wine has been consumed. This is the reason alcohol should not be drunk on an empty stomach, as an aperitif for example or during the course of the morning or afternoon.

When we drink wine whilst eating, the enzyme ADH in the stomach gets a chance to act and metabolise the alcohol over a period of time, ensuring that it does not increase too rapidly and cause problems to the system. Even if we only drink a glass of wine, it is important to eat first. The pylorus at the far end of the stomach should be stimulated to close by eating protein foods like roasted peanuts, olives, cheese, slices of pure meat sausage like salami, smoked salmon or surimi. Biscuits or crisps on the other hand, will not have the same effect.

At the same time it should be borne in mind that there are significant variations in the amount of gastric ADH produced:

- women produce half the amount produced by men, which undoubtedly explains why they cope less well with alcohol than do men

- Asiatics produce 85% less than their European counterparts. This is also the case with peoples like the Inuit, Native Americans or the Aborigines of Australia, who have lived for thousands of years on the fringes of our civilisation.

It is suggested that groups of humans who have traditionally consumed little or no alcohol during the course of their history have not developed the enzyme ADH necessary to metabolise it. For this reason they are more liable to become drunk and also to become alcoholics.

In the case of alcoholics in Western countries, it has been noticed that their level of gastric ADH is 50% lower than average and sometimes is totally non-existent. These factors must surely contribute substantially to the chronic nature of their illness.

144

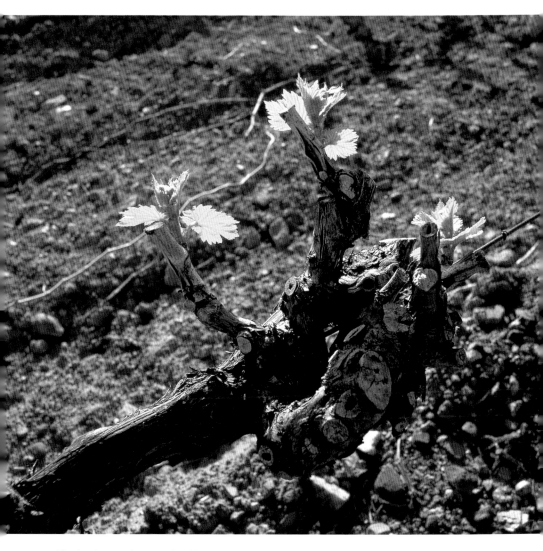

The first leaves of spring – late March in the vineyard at La Londe-les-Maures, Var, France.

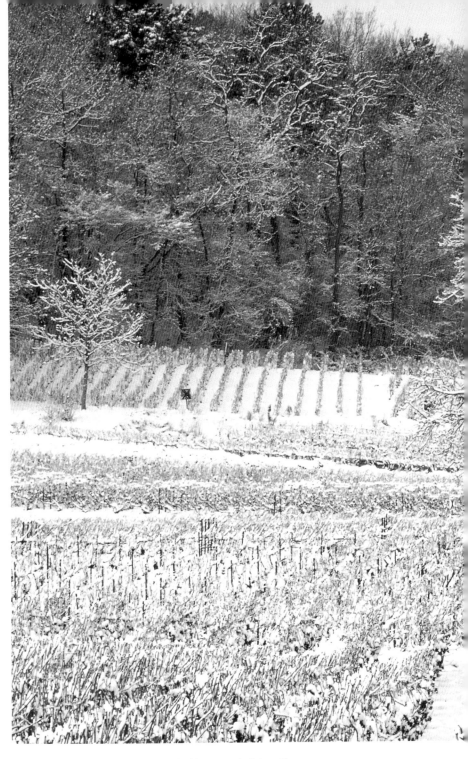

Snow blankets a vineyard at Verzy on the Montagne de Reims, France.

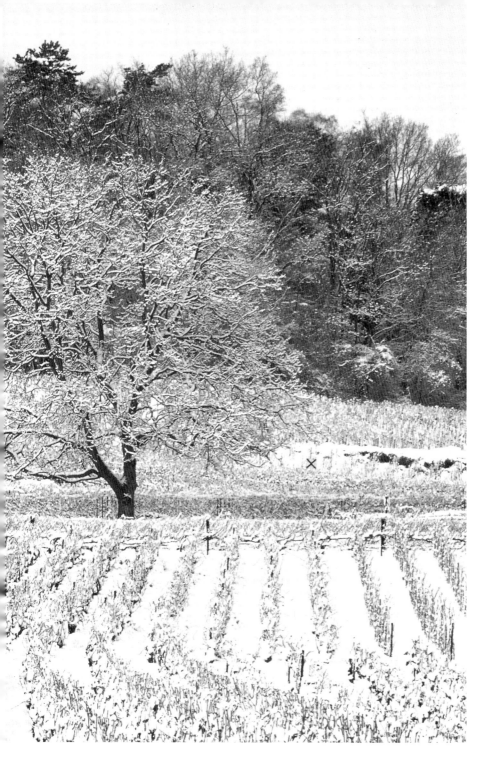

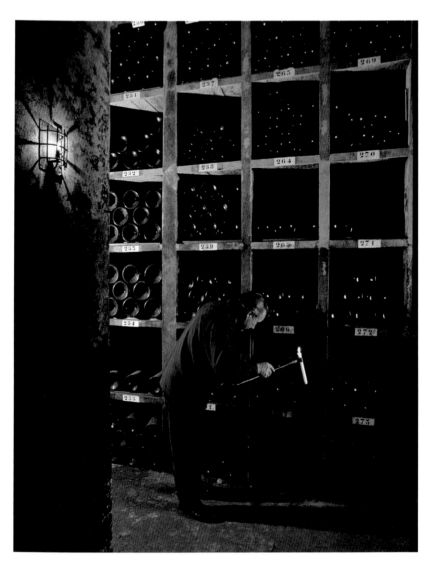

Mr. Jean Malbec, the Maitre de Chai of Chateau Latour, examines a Jeroboam of 1983 in the vintage bottle cellar.   *Chateau Latour, Pauillac, France.*

Certain medicines (anti-H2) often prescribed for treating ulcers of the stomach or duodenum, can also impede the action of gastric ADH either partially or even totally.

The pernicious effects of alcohol excess on the metabolism

Glycaemia

An excessive consumption of alcohol (particularly of whisky, gin, vodka or rum) on an empty stomach and not followed by a meal, can lead to hypoglycaemia – a condition where the level of glucose in the blood falls below its normal level of 1gm per litre of blood.

With alcohol blocking neoglucogenesis, there will be a lack of glucose in the blood and glycaemia will thus have a tendency to fall. If this drop is progressive, the following symptoms will become apparent: headaches, yawning, tiredness, lack of concentration, loss of memory, impaired vision, feelings of coldness and irritability.

If the wine drunk on an empty stomach is also sweet (like Pineau, Port, Sauternes, Sangria) secondary hypoglycaemia is likely to be more severe. In extreme cases, the condition of hypoglycaemia can be quite dramatic, with outbreaks of sweating, palpitations and trembling, accompanied by feelings of severe hunger and anxiety – which can become so bad, the sufferer loses consciousness.

Diabetes

If wine is drunk during a meal, it will not destabilise those who are insulin dependent, so long as they do not drink more than two glasses of wine per meal. More than that, and the diabetic will be at risk.

However, if the wine is taken on an empty stomach, the chance of hypoglycaemia occurring – often without any warning – is high.

With a diabetic Type II non-insulin dependent, two glasses of wine taken during the course of meals will more likely than not, improve glucose tolerance and thus lower the level of glycaemia. This beneficial effect is due to an improvement in the sensitivity to insulin and to the soluble fibres in wine that will reduce the absorption of carbohydrates consumed during the meal.

More than two glasses of wine will on the other hand, lead to an increase in hyperinsulinism and subsequently to insulin resistance.

Furthermore, it should be noted that alcoholism leads to an intolerance to glucose, which can lead to diabetes. Over half of chronic alcoholics have an intolerance to glucose and statistics show that 10% of cirrhosis sufferers have diabetes, as opposed to 4% of the population as a whole.

The muscular system

In the case of excessive consumption of wine, there is a significant risk of losing muscular mass since amino acids derived from protein are absorbed with difficulty by the small intestine.

The immune system

An excess of alcohol leads to a drop in the level of albumin in the blood – a sign that the body is undernourished and the immune system is weakened, making the person more vulnerable to infection.

The cardiovascular system

We have seen in Chapter 6 that moderate consumption of wine (2 to 4 glasses a day) had a beneficial effect on cholesterol levels, a lowering of overall cholesterol levels including "bad" LDL-cholesterol and an increase of "good" HDL-cholesterol.

However, with an increased consumption – bearing in mind individual sensitivities – the level of triglycerides can reach critical levels. Regular heavy doses of wine (4 to 5 glasses per meal) can lead to an excessive quantity of free radicals being produced, which is not counterbalanced by the positive action of polyphenols.

Besides this, an excessive consumption of wine can lead to an increased risk of high blood pressure, particularly with red wine. The 'J-type' curve, which translates the relationship between the two, shows that the lowest blood pressure results from the consumption of 2 glasses of wine: over 5 glasses, the maximum and minimum increase by 10 mm of mercury per extra glass.

The effect of alcohol on blood pressure only shows itself after 24 or 48 hours and then disappears providing no further alcohol is drunk. This explains the high blood pressure suffered on a Monday morning by people who have drunk heavily over the weekend and the fact that by the following Friday their blood pressure is normal again.

The incidence of high blood pressure is two or three times higher among heavy drinkers than among those that drink moderately. Alcohol excess is second only to obesity as a cause of high blood pressure and among heavy drinkers, one in four suffers from high blood pressure.

We know, of course, that high blood pressure increases the risk of heart attacks and strokes, but excessive alcohol consumption can cause other cardiovascular problems:

- *Cardio-myopathic obstructions* – ventricular problems leading to a change of circulation in the heart

- *Abnormalities in cardiac rhythm* – these account for 17% of deaths in those under 50 years of age

- *Cardiac insufficiency* resulting in breathlessness during effort or even when asleep. In extreme cases, severe water retention (oedemas) can occur in the legs.

- *Cerebrovascular accidents (strokes)* are the third most important cause of death in France and the prime cause of chronic invalidity.

There are two types of cerebrovascular accidents, which are differentiated by their mechanisms:

Ischaemic – these are cerebral thromboses caused by the obstruction of an artery in the brain and we have seen that this risk is substantially reduced by the moderate daily consumption of wine (2 to 4 glasses per day). On the other hand, consuming more than 6 glasses a day can substantially increase the risk.

Haemorrhagic – these result from the rupture of blood vessels in the brain brought about by blood pressure.

The anticlotting action of wine can lead to haemorrhages and excessive consumption of wine can aggravate this anticlotting action. Elderly people suffering with high blood pressure should therefore be advised to drink wine with moderation.

The digestive system

THE STOMACH

Drinking too much wine can result in a reflux of stomach acids towards the oesophagus where inflammation and lesions (oesophagites) can occur.

THE LIVER

Drinking more than 7 or 8 glasses of wine per day on a regular basis will encourage fatty deposits to build up progressively in the liver (hepatic steatosis). Among these heavy drinkers, one in two will suffer alcoholic hepatitis. The alcohol reaching the liver (acetaldehyde) in large quantities becomes toxic forming free radicals, which oxidise the liver cells and inhibit the regeneration of the hepatic cellular structure.

When hepatitis occurs, the lesions are reversible after a few weeks of abstinence. However, after 10 or 20 years of intemperance, 10% of heavy drinkers will develop cirrhosis, which is irreversible. This will be accompanied by changes in the immune system, allowing antibodies to form in the body, which will attack the liver of the patient and attempt to destroy it. Cirrhosis then becomes an autoimmune illness.

Bearing in mind that a woman produces less of the enzyme ADH, if she then drinks a litre of wine a day, she will run 35 times more risk of having cirrhosis than a man.

It is difficult for a doctor to diagnose these lesions if the patient does not admit to excessive drinking habits, as the symptoms are fairly common: lack of appetite, loss of weight, morning sickness and an increase of transaminase (a liver enzyme) in the blood.

The gall bladder

When more than 4 or 5 glasses of wine are drunk during a meal, the gall bladder may not contract normally, resulting sometimes in a poor digestion of fats in the small intestine and an abnormal stagnation of bile in the organ, leading eventually to the formation of gall stones in some patients.

The level of uric acid

The accumulation of lactic acid in the body after consuming large amounts of alcohol will result in less uric acid being eliminated through the kidneys.

High levels of uric acid (more than 70 mg/l) is often a sign of chronic alcoholism and can lead to an unexpected attack of gout when drinking a large quantity of wine. The risk is greatest when drinking Burgundies and least when drinking Champagne.

The endocrine glands

It has been noticed that alcoholic men suffer with impaired testicular function, resulting in a reduction in the level of testosterone and a relative increase in the level of oestrogen. This leads to the following side effects:

- An increase in the volume of the breasts (gynaecomastia) in 19% of the cases examined

- A reduction in hair growth

- Obesity in the lower body (of the gynoidal type)

- Red spots on the skin, particularly on the face and hands

- Impotence with libido problems associated with 40% of cases

- Absence of ejaculation in 80% of the cases when sexual activity is still possible. As the proverb says: "Bacchus is the enemy of Venus."

Women can have problems in ovulating if they drink more than five glasses of wine per day. In fact, sterility is three times more frequent among women drinking five glasses a day and six times more frequent with women that drink more than six glasses a day.

On the other hand, the temporary increase in the level of testosterone in women when consuming a substantial amount of wine may have an aphrodisiac effect that could explain some sexual behaviour patterns when under the influence of alcohol. It also explains why some men will try and seduce a woman by giving her too much to drink!

149

The assimilation of micronutrients

VITAMINS

The normal supply of vitamins is insufficient to meet the requirements of an alcoholic:

- *Owing to reduced intake* – an alcoholic eats little and is therefore undernourished at a time when his need for vitamin B1 has increased in order to produce the enzyme ALDH which is essential for metabolising alcohol.
- *Owing to reduced absorption through the intestine*
- *Owing to reduced liver function* – since the liver frequently intervenes in the assimilation of vitamins by the body
- *Owing to the increased loss of vitamins in the urine.*

Vitamin deficiency is an important factor as far as alcoholics are concerned, contributing to the toxic effect of alcohol, particularly at the neurological level.

MINERALS

High levels of alcohol in the bloodstream reduce the absorption of calcium through the small intestine and therefore contribute to osteoporosis, particularly in the case of women.

The alcoholic is also often deficient in phosphorus. Firstly, this is because the supply of nutrients is insufficient, and then because lesions contribute to a loss of phosphorus from the kidneys in the urine and finally because the level of magnesium in the blood is low.

This lack of phosphorus leads to psychological and neurological problems: irritability, disorientation, tingling in the arms and legs, difficulties in expressing oneself and even convulsions.

TRACE ELEMENTS

Excessive consumption of wine can have two different consequences: either a deficiency in trace elements or an excess.

A lack of zinc is responsible for:

- The malfunction of the gonads (testicles and ovaries)
- Problems with night vision
- Immune deficiencies leading to infections.

A lack of selenium contributes to a weakening in the number of anti-oxidants destined to fight against free radicals. By contrast, the level of lead is increased in the blood of the immoderate wine drinker as well as the level of iron that can contribute to the fixing of free radicals.

Alcohol excess and neurological troubles

Increase in headaches

Hypersensitive people can have headaches as a result of drinking wine. This is due to the various chemical substances to be found in it in varying quantities: histamine, tyramine, but particularly sulphites and sometimes methanol.

Risk of ear, nose and throat disorders

An excessive consumption of wine over a long period (20 to 30 years) can lead to auditory problems (34% of those unable to differentiate sounds) and problems of balance due to lesions to the inner ear (in 45% of cases). The problems of balance can also be due to lesions of the cerebellum. In effect, the cells of the cerebellar cortex are partially destroyed by drinking too much alcohol.

Effect on the nerves

The lack of vitamin B1 and the toxic action of alcohol itself, are conducive to lesions in the neurones which can result in inflammatory lesions of the nerves. These manifest themselves in difficulties with walking, in visual disorders and violent pains.

Effect on vigilance

A slight level of alcohol in the blood of between 0.3 gm/l and 0.5 gm/l is accompanied by a feeling of well being and euphoria. However, when the level exceeds 1gm/l, drowsiness sets in.

One or two glasses of wine at dinner can help to increase the length of nocturnal sleep. On the other hand, if these amounts are increased significantly, the opposite happens and it becomes difficult to fall asleep, the periods of deep slow sleep are reduced and REM sleep is increased.

Besides this, alcohol taken in excessive quantities modifies pulmonary ventilation during the night, leading to a possible apnoea or the cessation of breathing while the person is asleep. This phenomenon is more likely when obesity is associated with the condition, and the interruptions to the breathing pattern lead to poor oxygenation of the blood and feelings of intense tiredness upon waking.

Psychological disorders associated with alcohol excess

Raised levels of alcohol in the blood lead to behavioural problems:

- Drunkenness (loss of balance, mental confusion)
- Aggressive behaviour
- Bouts of delirium (obsessions, fixations, persecution complexes)
- Convulsions and even epileptic fits.

Deprived of alcohol due to hospitalisation or imprisonment, impressive disorders can occur, such as *delirium tremens,* characterised by severe shaking and hallucinations.

With the average chronic alcoholic, disorders are more difficult to interpret since they seem to be more a question of degree, with:

- Behavioural changes (irritability, instability, impulsiveness, frequent bouts of anger, physical and verbal abuse to family and friends)
- Emotional instability, with alternating bouts of intense excitement and severe depression
- Feelings of jealousy towards a partner or towards colleagues
- Persistent fixations.

152

Unfortunately, the best means for the alcoholic to bring matters under control is, paradoxically, to drink more alcohol.

The interaction between wine and medicines

Inhibitory effects

Some medicines have the effect of inhibiting the enzyme ALDH, leading to a build-up of acetaldehyde (incompletely metabolised alcohol). This can be translated into nausea, vomiting, a redness of the face and feelings of vertigo.

A certain number of medicines have this effect, particularly:

- Sulpha drugs inducing hypoglycaemia, used in Type II Diabetes

- Some fungicides prescribed to treat mycoses

- Some antibiotics (cephalosporines).

The patient should therefore be warned of these possible side effects if wine is drunk whilst taking medication. In the case of the alcoholic, since it is unlikely he or she will abstain from alcohol, then they should ask the doctor for alternative medicines.

The interference between medicines and alcohol

The action of medicines can vary considerably if the patient is a heavy drinker:

- If the metabolism of the liver is activated in order to cope with alcohol in the form of acetaldehyde, then medication is available more quickly to the system and in higher concentrations. If this is the case, there is a real risk of the medication poisoning the body or aggravating the side effects of the treatment, inducing severe drowsiness for example.

- If the liver is unable to cope with the medicine whilst metabolising the alcohol, then the concentration of medicine too weak and the treatment is correspondingly less effective.

The list of medications that interfere with alcohol is very long, but doctors are well equipped to determine which medicines are most suited to the needs of their patients.

Below is a list of difficult medicines that need to be watched:

- Antiepileptics, that are often prescribed to alcoholics.

- Tranquillisers and anxiolitics, whose effects are increased when taken with alcohol in the body. The main risk is acute drowsiness, which can be very dangerous if the patient attempts to drive a car. The memory can also be affected, leading in some instances to amnesia whilst the patient is on medication.

- Certain bensodiazepine taken with alcohol can produce behavioural disorders (aggression and lack of inhibition) which have sometimes resulted in the patients committing crimes of which they have no recollection. Taking these medicines can be accompanied by total memory loss that can last for several hours.

- Mixing alcohol and antihistamine drugs (prescribed for allergic reactions) or alcohol and certain analgesics (prescribed to suppress pain) is very dangerous if driving a car since only a small amount of alcohol (less than 0.5 mg/l) is required to bring about acute drowsiness. It is important therefore to read very carefully indeed any warnings associated with medicines.

It is useful to know that coffee taken at the end of a meal accompanied by alcohol has the effect of slowing down the rate at which the stomach empties itself. The level of alcohol in the blood may therefore be lower at that moment, but the level and the effects will persist longer. So if you want to drive the car fairly shortly after this type of meal, it is better not to drink coffee.

Former alcoholics who have stopped drinking and who take medication to help them resist temptation, should be very careful when prescribed different medicines, as some may contain alcohol. This is rarely a problem in the United Kingdom, but those who live in France should beware of the following:

- *Some tonics:* Acti 5, Activarol, Ascencyl, Debrumyl, Revitalose C 1000, Surelen, natural Cortine among others

154

- *Some cough syrups:* Terpine Gonnon among others

- *Some sedatives:* Euphytose, Passiflorine, Phytocalm among others

- *Some herbal or homeopathic medicines taken in drops.*

The carcinogenic effect of alcohol

We saw in Chapter 7 that if we drink wine rich in polyphenols on a daily basis and in moderation, we will benefit from the antioxidising action of the flavinoids, which will have a powerful inhibiting effect on free radicals, thus protecting us from cancer.

However, this phenomenon is reversed when the quantity of alcohol increases: the action of the polyphenols is inadequate to stop the formation of free radicals induced by alcohol excess. Excessive consumption of wine on a regular basis increases the risk of cancers developing in the mouth, tongue, pharynx, larynx, oesophagus, liver, rectum, bladder and breast.

Alcohol is not necessarily carcinogenic in itself. It is probably only carcinogenic when it acts in concert with other cancer forming substances, helping them to penetrate the gut by damaging the cells of the small intestine.

However, some alcohols can act as carriers for carcinogenic compounds. In a study published in 1996, Kleinjans showed that whiskies contained quantities of benzopyrenes, which varied according to the care taken in their preparation. Paradoxically the most ordinary whiskies, and thus the least refined and the cheapest, were also the least dangerous.

An excess of alcohol increases the level of cytochrome P450 in the liver, which is known to turn certain substances in the body cancerous. Moreover, some alcoholic drinks sometimes contain carcinogenic substances (nitrosamines in beer and benzopyrenes in cider) that are helped by alcohol to penetrate the intestinal wall.

Wine is not implicated in cancers of the bladder, only drinks made of aniseed, though it should be borne in mind that alcohol abuse leads to an immune deficiency, which in turn leads to cancers. However, in the field of cancers, the most dangerous synergy is that of alcohol and

155

tobacco. This combination dramatically increases the risk of cancers occurring in the upper respiratory and alimentary tracts. For instance, the risk of a person contracting cancer if they smoked 30 cigarettes and drank one litre of wine per day, is increased by a factor of 87. If the same person drank a further two alcoholic drinks, such as whisky or aniseed, the risk factor would be increased to 150.

Wine and pregnancy

We have seen that alcoholics have an increased risk of sterility due to lesions in the gonads. Furthermore, alcohol is a problem as soon as fertilisation occurs and it involves not only the mother but also the father. If the mother does not drink but the father does – and to excess – there will be no morphological abnormalities. On the other hand, there will be the risk of cerebral abnormality leading to intellectual and behavioural problems, possibly caused by lesions to the spermatazoa, which in turn can lead to abnormal replication of RNA (ribonucleic acid) caused by problems with protein synthesis.

The risk of having more obvious disorders is increased if the mother herself has an abnormal consumption of alcohol at the time of conception. This is why, as soon as a woman suspects she may be pregnant, she should drink little or no wine or alcohol. For women who drink more than four glasses of wine a day, the risk of miscarriage increases by 17%.

What then is the daily amount of wine that a pregnant woman can take without endangering the foetus?

One glass of wine a day appears to have no adverse effect. Two to four glasses a day increases the risk of malformation in 10% of cases and the birth weight in most cases was below average. It is known that alcohol passes easily across the placenta into the blood circulation of the foetus. There is also a risk of cerebral lesions that may result in a lower than average IQ at the age of four.

In the case of a pregnant mother drinking more than five to six glasses of wine per day, which is excessive, the chances of the foetus manifesting the following malformations associated with a foeto-alcoholic syndrome is put at about 50% :

156

- A forehead with abnormal protrusion

- An exaggerated distance between nose and top lip

- A harelip

- A small receding chin

- Delayed growth (weight and height)

- Minor disorders of the heart, kidneys, bone structure and male genitalia.

In France, this syndrome exists in a minor form in 4 to 5 births per 1,000 and in serious form in 1 to 2 births per 1,000.

Among the children affected, it is possible to observe a delay in learning to walk at 18 months. However, these children can also suffer with hyperactivity, poor concentration and lethargic reactions.

At the age of 10 to 13, the IQ of these children is lower than average and 61% of the boys as well as 17% of the girls still suffer from stunted growth.

The greatest risk of this foeto-alcoholic syndrome developing is at the time of conception, and during the first and fifth months of pregnancy.

But in 85% of the cases, alcoholic excess is associated with a nicotine and caffeine dependency as well.

Wine and breastfeeding

If a mother who is breastfeeding drinks alcohol, 1.7% of the alcohol absorbed into her system passes into her milk. This translates into about 84 milligrams of alcohol per litre of breast milk if the mother drinks one or two glasses of wine per day.

This amount may appear derisorily small, but it is important because the infant does not yet have the enzymes (HAD in particular) necessary to oxidise this alcohol which otherwise will go directly to the brain. When this happens, there will be behavioural disorders and particularly a disruption to the time set aside for sleep.

Furthermore, breast milk containing alcohol has a specific smell that

157

the infant dislikes. As a result, the feeding time will tend to be shorter as a result and the child will run the risk of being undernourished. To exacerbate the problem further, the nipple will be not be stimulated sufficiently and this will result in less milk being produced.

Reasons enough for the mother who breastfeeds, to abstain totally from alcohol if she can.

CHAPTER 9

ALCOHOLISM

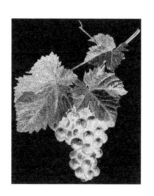

We have seen in the last chapter what the consequences may be for our health if we drink too much wine and alcohol. With a heavy drinker, wines and more particularly beer and spirits are in fact drunk together and it is difficult to determine exactly how much alcohol has been taken into the body.

At what point can you start talking about alcoholism? Alcoholism is present when the drinker becomes alcohol-dependent. Then alcohol becomes a drug: the drinker is no longer able to live without alcohol and has lost the power to abstain. The alcoholic can think of little else and will resort to any subterfuge to satisfy his craving.

There are not many alcoholics who are exclusively wine drinkers. In France, they are normally tramps who over indulge in low-grade wine because it is the cheapest way of getting drunk. However, wine alcoholics are also present in rural areas, even if they are something of a disappearing race. This is because drinking wine throughout the day has always been a part of country life – perhaps even an obligation. Barely 30 years ago, "having a postman's nose" still meant a person looked the worse for drink. This expression came into being because country postmen were practically obliged to drink a glass of wine at every farm where they delivered the mail.

Nowadays, about two-thirds of alcoholism is linked to the consumption of beer and hard spirits like gin, whisky, vodka and brandy. Mainly wine drinkers make up the remaining third.

THE SYMPTOMS

When a person suddenly gives up drinking alcohol, the physical and psychological disorders which follow may reveal an unsuspected dependency. Symptoms of physical dependency will manifest themselves in perspiration, nausea, tachycardia (when the heart races), insomnia or "the morning shakes". These signs that testify to a body craving alcohol will disappear in a few minutes after the patient has taken 10 to 20 grams of alcohol.

Psychological dependency will become apparent when there are signs of anxious behaviour, a lack of emotional stability and aggression brought about by a fixation, almost an obsession, to satisfy the urge to drink.

A medical diagnosis is not always easy, because the patient rarely talks about his problem when he visits the doctor about symptoms that are common to other pathologies – like problems with digestion, hypertension, anxiety, irritability, depression, impotence and cramp. However, there are certain signs that can point the doctor in the right direction: a bloated face that is abnormally coloured and blotchy, a particular smell to the breath or trembling at the extremities. Laboratory tests will also confirm his diagnosis and particularly:

- *Gamma GT levels:* the increased levels of this enzyme in heavy drinkers was discovered in 1972. The normal amount found in blood serum is below 36 IU in men and 25 IU in women. However, it is not a very reliable indicator, since 40% of alcoholics can have a normal level, while 13% of those that are not alcoholics can have a level which is too high. High levels of Gamma GT can in fact be ascribed to other conditions – including the taking of medicines

- *Average corpuscular volume:* with heavy drinkers, the size of red blood corpuscles increases (macrocytosis), although this condition can result from a deficiency of vitamins B9 and B12 during pregnancy and as a result of thyroid problems

- *The level of triglycerides:* it is only excessive in 30% of those cases that have high levels of alcohol in their blood. Comparison between clinical indicators and analysis of the blood will allow the doctor to be more precise with his diagnosis.

ALCOHOLISM IN FRANCE

The total amount of alcohol consumed in France has declined quite sharply over the last 30 years – by about 34% – though the number of heavy drinkers has remained unchanged. As we shall see later on, alcoholism is a terrible illness that is a long way from being overcome. However, France is not unique in facing this sad situation, since most other countries share the same problem.

Out of 58 million French people, statistics show us that 7 million (12% of the population) are heavy drinkers, 2½ million are alcohol dependent (of which 900,000 are women) and 78,000 are officially recognised as alcoholics and are under the care of Social Security, classified with those suffering from "long term illnesses". Each year, alcoholism costs the country 80 billion francs in medical care – about 9 billion pounds sterling – and the life expectancy of an alcoholic is twelve years less than the average. Alcoholism accounts for nearly 10% of all deaths in France, each year.

Causes of death among alcoholics

%	Cause
28%	Cirrhosis
25%	Lung and stomach cancers
16%	Traffic accidents
9%	Domestic and sporting accidents
7%	Serious complications (haemorrhages, comas)
7%	Suicides
2.5%	Murders
2%	Tuberculosis
1.5%	Accidents at work

Studies conducted on alcoholics show that the risk is inversely proportional to the level of achievement in education and in social and professional spheres. More than 70% of alcoholics failed to take the French equivalent of GCE "A" levels and 30% did not even receive secondary education. Moreover, 55% of alcoholics are out of work.

Number of glasses of alcohol consumed daily by alcoholics (wine, beer and spirits)

27%	Less than 5 glasses
23%	Between 5 and 9 glasses
34%	Between 10 and 19 glasses
12%	Between 20 to 29 glasses
4%	30 glasses and over

HEREDITY AND ALCOHOLISM

Since the time of Ancient Greece, it has been thought likely that heredity, particularly through the mother, could be a risk factor with regard to alcoholism. Aristotle stated that "alcoholic women give birth to children like themselves". Plutarch observed that "one alcoholic gives birth to another".

Since then, many studies have been made and it has always been difficult to determine the extent to which family environment or social context has contributed to heavy drinking. The results from these studies and conclusions that followed from them are as follows:

- Regarding family influence, it has been shown that having an alcoholic parent multiplies the risk of becoming alcoholic by a factor of five in the case of men, and a factor of four in the case of women.

- In the studies conducted on twins by Kaïg, it has been shown that if one of the twins is alcoholic, the other has a 54% chance of being alcoholic if they are identical twins as compared to a 29% chance with fraternal twins.

- In studies conducted on adopted children, men ran an 18% risk of being alcoholic if one of their biological parents was alcoholic, whereas the risk was only 4% if their biological parents were not alcoholic.

Overall, the majority of the studies shows that heredity definitely plays a part in alcoholism, particularly in the case of men. In 1994, Fumeron identified a gene that could play a role in the excessive consumption of alcohol, as well as engender obesity and drug addiction. Thus, the child of an alcoholic would have a much higher risk of becoming an abuser of alcohol, drugs or food (sugar, for instance).

Alcoholism has a definite hereditary component, though not necessarily an automatic one. However, it is always difficult to differentiate between an inborn and an external influence in these matters, since environmental factors appear to play such a significant role. In fact, one could say that heredity predisposes by contributing to a higher vulnerability. Later, environment proposes and finally, the personality of the individual disposes and triumphs.

A person with alcoholic parents is therefore not doomed to alcohol dependence. For this to develop, the person in question needs to be confronted by psychological factors which are difficult to cope with and will act as a trigger.

THE MECHANISM OF ALCOHOL DEPENDENCY

It is possible to ask oneself whether an excessive consumption of alcohol is merely a bad habit or whether it is linked to a real dependence, as for example in the case of drugs.

A drug leads to a tolerance on the one hand and dependence accompanied by withdrawal symptoms on the other. With an alcoholic there is also an alcoholic tolerance: some people can consume between 200 and 300 grams of alcohol a day (20 to 30 glasses), whereas the average person would be in a deep coma long before they drank this amount of alcohol.

With a true alcoholic, these levels of alcohol in the blood do not necessarily preclude living more-or-less normally. Perhaps he is not acutely aware of what is going on, but we should not forget that 85% of fatal accidents caused by people under the influence of alcohol whilst driving are caused by people who only drink occasionally. The hardened alcoholic is responsible for a mere 15%, which would seem to show that they are better able to cope with the destabilising effects of alcohol.

165

The brain has shown itself to be quite capable of adapting itself to its new alcoholic environment, though this is not in the patient's interest because he or she will always pride themselves on being able to hold their drink. This is where the real problem lies; for in developing this tolerance, the alcoholic suppresses the disagreeable effects of alcohol that could have acted as a warning against excess.

The World Health Organisation officially defined dependency in 1975 as: "A psychological and sometimes physical state, resulting from the interaction between a living organism and a substance, characterised by behavioural responses which always include a compulsion (an irresistible impulse to realise and act contrary to the will and reason) to take and consume the substance continually or periodically to gain psychological effects and sometimes avoid the discomfort associated with withdrawal."

This official definition of dependency is very interesting, because it is not centred on the substance as is the definition of drug taking. Rather it focuses on the link between the substance (alcohol in this case) and the subject (the alcoholic). In other words, we do not look at the ball dragged by the alcoholic but at his chain.

With such a definition, dependence is not associated with the product but with the inability of the person to do without it, which enables us to qualify the subject as alcoholic. With this notion of dependency, the product becomes a prop. It may not even exist: the people who cannot stop playing at the casino or gamble at the races and the compulsive shopper, act in a similar way to the drug addict – but without the drug. Whatever the cost, these people are in search of a pleasure that has enslaved them. Besides which, the success rates after three months of trying to break the habit, are strangely similar to those recorded for both tobacco and heroin.

Comparative success rates for overcoming addiction to heroin, alcohol and tobacco (after Hunt)

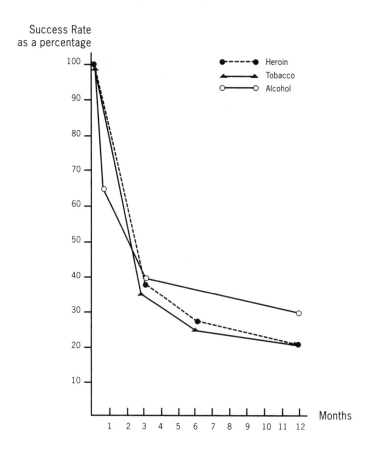

Physical dependency

A part of our brain makes conscious decisions linked to the will. For the sake of convenience, I will call this the voluntary brain. It decides on a certain number of actions that are implemented through a conscious and desired movement. But there is also a part of our brain, which regulates many functions outside our voluntary control (the rhythm of the heart and lungs, oxygen deficiency, heat balance, digestive and hormonal secretions and so on). For the sake of convenience again, I will call this the automatic brain.

The role of the automatic brain

If our body is in a state of hypoglycaemia (with a low sugar level in the blood), our automatic brain is presented with a strong feeling of hunger. This will trigger an urge to seek and consume food, which will be difficult to repress.

When the stomach is full, we then enter a period of satiety that will last until a new feeling of hunger appears. This perpetual oscillation between a "lack" and an "excess" (or sufficiency) is the basis of all regulating systems.

Drinking follows the same pattern: the alcoholic does not feel well unless he or she has a certain level of alcohol in the blood. When this begins to go down because the effects of the last glass are declining, the alcoholic will need a new supply of alcohol to suppress his withdrawal symptoms – or feeling deprived of alcohol. Gradually the automatic brain will take over control of the level of alcohol in the blood, as it controls the level of oxygen, the level of glucose and body temperature.

The regulatory systems are similar to the movements of a pendulum. As far as food is concerned, an internal pendulum periodically reminds us that if we do not eat, we will die. Eating pushes the pendulum away and our pangs of hunger disappear, but a few hours later inexorably the pendulum returns to reawaken our desire to eat.

This image of the pendulum suits the alcoholic very well: the periodic return of the need to drink alcohol. As we have seen, the body eventually regulates the level of alcohol in the blood with the result that with the person dependent on alcohol, in addition to the vital messages like "if you do not breathe, you die", "if you do not eat, you die", there is the additional refrain "if you do not drink alcohol, you die"! As a result, each time the level of alcohol in the blood falls, it has to be increased regardless of cost, in defiance of will and in defiance of reason. It is as if the automatic brain has included alcohol among those elements that are essential for life.

The automatic brain acts like a robot. However, the voluntary brain does not struggle against it on an equal footing, because the automatic brain has been at work twenty-four hours a day since the day we were born. The will is powerless against this physical dependency. Dependency is not due solely to the level of alcohol in the blood. Far from it. Many other chemical substances are involved in explaining it.

Biological factors

SEROTONIN is a neuro-transmitter that has many psychological effects on blood circulation and sexual behaviour, on sleep and particularly on depression. With the alcoholic there is an increase in the capture of serotin by blood platelets. As a result, there is a reduction in the concentration of serotonin at the junction between the neurones – the synapses – which is the direct consequence of an increased consumption of alcohol.

FREE RADICALS are made when there is too much alcohol in the blood and they alter the fatty membranes of the cerebral neurones through a process of peroxidation. These membrane changes make the nerve cells less adaptable. When alcohol is eliminated from the body, they are unable to readapt quickly to the new physiological conditions and withdrawal symptoms appear.

DOPAMINE is secreted by the neurones in the meso-cortico-limbic area of the brain and it has been shown that they are implicated in the evolution and maintenance of drug taking. Like nicotine, cannabis, morphine or cocaine, alcohol is capable of activating neurones. Thus a reward system from the brain comes into play. This dopamine "pleasure-giving" is also activated by natural stimuli like food, novelty or sex. On the other hand, when drinking stops, a lack of dopamine activity leads to withdrawal symptoms and a quest for intoxicants.

If alcohol is drunk repeatedly to avoid the disagreeable experiences associated with withdrawal, the more often alcohol will be taken because is releases the "pleasure shots" similar to those released by opiates. This pleasure reinforces the imprinting of behavioural patterns that will result in the loss of free choice and voluntary command over behaviour.

On their own, none of these biochemical mechanisms can be respon-sible for the development of phenomena as complex as dependence and tolerance. It is certain that several of them come into play and act together.

Genetic factors

These were dealt with at the beginning of this chapter.

Factors pertaining to character

The following personality traits, found particularly in adolescents, tend to favour dependency:

- A rebellious child, badly controlled and hostile to its mother

- Extrovert behaviour

- Impulsiveness or aggression

- Poor concentration (perhaps in childhood the subject was unstable and hyperactive)

- Social immaturity with predisposition to phobias (alcohol would then help to relieve inhibitions)

- Non-conformist social behaviour with an urge to transgress

- Obstinacy

- Desire to experience new things and strong sensations

- Indulgence towards one's own behaviour

- Intolerance of anxiety, depression and frustration

- Inability to tolerate the least conflict

- Dependence on rewards

- Affective immaturity, with oral regression ("food orgasm")

- An absence of narcissistic behaviour in childhood (alcohol will give access to feelings of over-riding power)

- Care in avoiding behaviour that causes hurt to others.

It should be stressed that these tendencies are not specific and do not automatically lead to alcohol abuse. As far as anxiety and depression are concerned, they are more the consequence of alcohol dependency rather than its cause.

Socio-cultural factors

The individual belongs to a group, to an ecological system, whose constraints determine the relationship of the individual to alcohol. But there is an interaction between the "demand" of the individual and the "supply" afforded by the environment.

The environment predisposes, but it is the person who disposes. Thus family environment, school environment, relationships with friends, military service and professional environment (where the individual is often exposed to regular consumption of alcoholic drinks) are all involved in the sociological factors that impinge on the individual.

Since alcohol can be strongly associated with pleasurable, convivial experiences – encounters with friends, family parties, hosting customers or participating in group ceremonies – it is easy to develop a behavioural dependency on alcohol.

As we recalled much earlier on, the consumption of alcohol in profane situations has its roots in the sacred use of wine. It is engraved in a cultural tradition that is particularly strong in France, where wine has traditionally been considered a "totem-drink".

But as wine has gradually come to be considered old-fashioned, Anglo-Saxon drinks suggesting greater virility have replaced it. Raising your glass has always been a profoundly symbolic act, but these days it has more worth if it is done with strong alcohol rather than with a glass of plonk. In France today, only the country peasant and the council road sweeper will raise their glass of wine to each other. Only Champagne is socially acceptable to the wider world.

Diagnosis of alcoholic dependency

It is not easy for the family of a person who drinks a lot of alcohol, to diagnose that that person is in fact alcohol-dependent. It is even more difficult for a doctor, because he has no reliable clinical guides.

However, there are certain indicators: if the person concerned drinks a lot, particularly spirits, and drinks frequently, then there is cause to be suspicious.

In one of the episodes in the French television serial *Navarro*, the famous superintendent is dealing with a young woman, whose inexperience as a magistrate leads her to charge a young drug addict with murder. The detective is more perceptive and is convinced of the young man's innocence. However, at this point he is so depressed that he takes refuge in the bar of his friend Ginou just as she is closing down for the night. Seeing her friend in this state and knowing his natural aversion to lemonade, Ginou hurries to serve him a glass of hard liquor like cognac or calvados. Having downed his glass in one go, Navarro says to his friend:

"Don't you have anything stronger?"

"Yes," she replies, "but I only use it to clean my windows!"

It has to be said, the characters drink a lot in this serial. Not only does one of the assistants – Inspector Auquelin – always have a flask of cognac about his person, but his chief superintendent Walts regularly takes a nip out of it as well. Each time that Navarro goes home, his professional job done, his daughter Yolande serves him with a large whisky, which he then drinks neat on an empty stomach.

Quite obviously this lifestyle is quite normal for Navarro. However, does it mean that he is an alcoholic? To answer this question it would be necessary to tot up how much he drinks during the course of the day: apparently several glasses of hard liquor (lets say two or three) but also wine – three good glasses at each meal, or the equivalent of a 75cl bottle. With a minimum daily intake of a bottle of wine and three glasses of spirit, Navarro is evidently a heavy drinker. However, to determine whether he is an alcoholic or not, it would be necessary to prevent him drinking for a couple of days and then observe how well he managed to cope just drinking mineral water. Probably not very well.

Since he is approaching 60 and we can imagine that he has been drinking like this for many years, it is likely that he would react badly to being weaned off alcohol and we would discover with surprise and disappointment that he is an alcoholic. Bearing in mind the risk factor that this presents for his health, we cannot but be afraid of what is in store for our favourite detective when he comes to retire, because there is every chance he will die prematurely. Either this, or he will suffer ill health for several years before finally he departs this mortal coil.

However, the case of Navarro is not unique. In the police force, probably to make the job more bearable, it would appear that there is a lot of heavy drinking. Here in France at least, where the writers make every attempt to stay as close to reality as possible, all the television series stress this point. Alcohol is shown as an indispensable support for the males of the species to fulfil their various roles. America has shown us for a long time, that the heroes of westerns, law-enforcing cowboys, sheriffs and marshals, would never have conquered the screen with a bottle of milk in their hands.

But apart from the French police (whose legendary dependency on alcohol is without doubt far more marginal today than it was in the past), there are numerous professions where it is customary rather than necessary to drink in order to be accepted within the group. Little by little, members of these professions are led to drink more than they should, increasing their alcohol resistance until finally they become alcohol dependent.

The dangers associated with hard liquor

Politeness, conviviality and social convention lead people to drink when they meet together. Social convention leads the host to offer their guests something to drink before they eat. Some years ago, the cup of friendship and the aperitif were celebrated with red or white wine, of varying quality and age depending on the social and cultural level – and particularly the economic level – of the group involved.

Today, in the majority of situations, wine is old fashioned. A certain snobbery has succeeded in replacing wine – whether it be red or white, dry, white, sweet or mulled – with drinks that come mainly from abroad. These days, it would not even cross the mind of a Frenchman to drink a cognac, armagnac or calvados as an aperitif. By contrast, whisky, gin or vodka, their close relations, are very welcome. Americans and particularly the Japanese, have no scruples in drinking French spirits as aperitifs. But whether they are foreign drinks or not, the result is the same: it is hard liquor, distilled alcohol in excess of 40° proof!

Drinking spirits on an empty stomach in the middle of the day (or night), is a deplorable habit for several reasons. Firstly, because it affects your metabolism and therefore your health, and as we have seen in Chapter 7, unlike wine which stimulates the gastric juices, hard liquor interferes quite fundamentally with their secretion. Secondly, because a generous quantity of whisky, gin or vodka contains enough alcohol to prevent you drinking anything else.

What tends to happen, however, is that spirit drinkers will drink a couple of large whiskies as an aperitif. When they and their friends ought to know that before sitting down to the table they will have already drunk more or less the alcoholic equivalent of a full bottle of wine. After which, of course, they will drink three, four, perhaps even five or six glasses of wine during the course of the meal, finishing off with another alcoholic drink at the end in the guise of a digestive.

If they happen to be a part of your group, bear in mind that they are in considerable danger. If they are occasional drinkers, not only do they run the risk of a heart attack when their body reacts, but they may very well wind up as one of the 85% that end up in a motor accident if they then happen to drive the car. Alternatively, if they are habitual drinkers, they are probably well on the road to becoming alcoholics – with all that that unfortunate state entails for their long-term health.

This is why we should do everything to change our social habits, drinking wine as an aperitif. If you have the financial means, drink champagne: if you are not that fortunate, then drink *crémants* or sparkling wines. Often they are just as good and two or three times cheaper.

THE TREATMENT OF ALCOHOLISM

In 1991, a survey conducted by IPSOS investigated the attitude of the public to alcoholism.

To the question: "In your opinion, is the excessive consumption of alcohol a weakness or an illness?" the answers were as follows:

51%	a weakness
43%	an illness
4%	no opinion
2%	either an accident of life or a lack of support

The same people interviewed were then asked what action in their opinion, was most likely to bring about an end of the condition. Their answers were as follows:

49%	the alcoholic should exercise will power
22%	friends should provide support
9%	the patient should go to Alcoholics Anonymous
4%	the patient should be referred to a doctor
2%	had no opinion
1%	the patient should be detoxified.

It emerged that the public had a completely wrong perception of what was wrong. The study of alcoholic dependence has shown that once the condition has developed, we are dealing with a real illness, which should be treated as such. What is more, there is a physical and pharmacological dependence, as well as a condition where the automatic brain has managed to dominate the voluntary brain. All of which make it quite unrealistic to think the problem can be overcome merely by appealing to will power.

This misunderstanding by the public of the mechanisms of dependency, as shown by this survey, constitutes a real problem because it is likely to result in a delay before the patient seeks specialist help. For a certain time, the alcoholic wrestles with the problem of his addiction. But in vain, because he seeks to control the uncontrollable. The automatic brain will always be stronger than the voluntary brain and failure will only reduce the individual's feelings of self esteem, which will be at a low ebb anyway.

But whom should you consult? The first step is for you to have the humility to recognise that alcohol is stronger than you are. Once this is clear, the best thing to do is to ask a specialist for help. This is always easier to do when you fully appreciate the nature of your condition. Go to a specialist used to dealing with these problems, who may be either a doctor or a psychologist, for too often ordinary practitioners have not received the specialist training needed to treat this complex condition.

What should the treatment offer? First and foremost there should be a full and frank discussion, conducted in an atmosphere of mutual trust. The therapist must explain to his patient that contrary to what is widely believed, alcoholism is not a vice but an illness needing treatment. To overcome it, the patient must understand the mechanisms of physical dependence, knowing that when confronted with physical dependence, the will plays no role in the treatment (which straight away should help the patient not to feel guilty for past failures).

The treatment should also offer psychological help. It is important the alcoholic should recover his self esteem, reinforce his "ego" and self regard. A cognitive and behavioural therapy will have to be put in place to alter the automatic responses and learn specifically how to manage abstinence when in a social situation. Above all, the motivation of the patient must not be based on fear of the consequences of alcoholism, but on the value of the benefits to be derived from breaking the habit.

In his book *Das Unbehagen in der Kultur*, Freud identified three ways in which man could find pleasure: work; creativity and drugs (alcohol, tobacco, cannabis, morphine). Since the alcoholic must rid himself of the drug component, he must learn how to channel his energy into another area. He must ask himself "what is it in life that fires me up sufficiently to give me the strength to break with this 'marvellous buddy' alcohol?".

It is important and even necessary to replace alcohol with something else. The alcoholic must find an aim in life. However, this positive and constructive step is not easy to accomplish on your own: despite good intentions, you run the risk of losing your nerve, all the more so because the traditional family is not much help in these circumstances. It is far better to seek out the support of former drinkers in organisations like Alcoholics Anonymous.

Giving up alcohol must be brutal and total. Not drinking means not pushing the pendulum anymore. And gradually, the need to drink will not come back. In this way, you manage to disconnect the automatic brain that stops feeling that drinking alcohol is essential for survival. The problem is the same with food: people on hunger strike, for example, notice that after a few days the feeling of hunger disappears. Weaning yourself away from alcohol can be done during detoxification treatment in a specialised clinic, but only if the patient expressly requests it. The therapist must not send the alcoholic there as an emergency without his consent. This brutal treatment of sending the patient into an unknown environment which is essentially hostile will subject him to stress which will be difficult to manage and may break the confidence between the therapist and his patient.

With the help of medication and good psychological support, weaning the alcoholic away from alcohol can be accomplished in town, without the need of going into hospital. However, it will require the patient to be absent from work for a few days. The medication is not very effective and cannot be used on its own to treat the alcoholic. However, they are an important part of the overall treatment that should last for at least a year.

Sadly, relapses are common. Unfortunately, the "call of alcohol" can always make itself heard because the biochemical changes to the body caused by alcoholism may persist for years. An alcoholic can therefore have a relapse at any time if he fails to abstain for the rest of his life. This is the reason it is almost impossible for a former alcoholic to become a moderate drinker, even if he has become psychologically reasonable. His body will always remain vulnerable.

From this we can conclude that the only real solution to this problem is prevention. At the end of the twentieth century, therapy cannot be content with caring for illness as it has done for the last 40 or 50 years. If it is to help make savings in the health service, it must organise a proper programme of prevention. Treating the patient means tertiary prevention: hopefully, by acting in time, we will thus avoid physical complications and early death.

Secondary prevention consists in tracking down people at risk, often already heavy drinkers but not yet alcohol dependent. Being vigilant and preventing people becoming alcoholics, is the task of the general practitioner. In some professions, trade unions are also involved in this field.

However, the main task is to bring into being a primary prevention – educating people about alcohol and giving the young an effective code of conduct in dealing with alcoholic drinks. Knowing how to drink is the best guarantee against alcoholism, which is still the cause of far too many deaths in our society today.

CHAPTER 10

Learning how to Drink

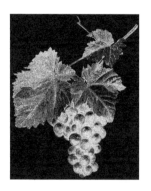

Just a few decades ago, the subject of sexuality was still taboo and puritanical attitudes were rife. Young girls from "good" families became pregnant without knowing what had happened to them and conscript soldiers discovered the venereal disadvantages of participating in civilian assault courses whilst on leave. The subject was not spoken about openly and useful advice, as well as bawdy jokes, were passed on in private.

More recently we have come to realise that the young should be properly informed if we want to try and contain unwanted pregnancies and sexually transmitted diseases. As a result, sex education has now been introduced into schools.

And what about education on the risks associated with food? What chance is there that children in schools will be given sound nutritional information when even doctors have received little or no education in this field? The subject has been ignored for so long by the faculties of medicine in most countries that, even today, nutritional information is mainly disseminated by the food industry, whose pearls of wisdom are often altered to suit their own commercial interests. Information about the consumption of alcoholic drinks has been handled so badly (or often not all) that the problem still remains a taboo subject – a subject that often provokes a misinformed and puritanical reaction.

The measures taken in a certain number of western countries – particularly France with its Evin law – bear witness to something that can best be described as neo-prohibition. For instead of attacking the real problem, which is an excessive consumption by the minority, they have succeeded in reducing the average consumption of wine by the majority. This consumption was relatively low in the first place.

In this way, we are presented by the strange and paradoxical situation. The greater number of reasonable drinkers drink less and less while the positive effects of moderate consumption have been made manifest by scientific research. The number of heavy drinkers, particularly alcoholics, remains the same, whilst alcoholic abuse by the young becomes an increasingly serious problem.

We shall succeed in achieving the real objectives of public health only if we concentrate on the dissemination of accurate information free from bias and out-dated prejudice.

THE YOUNG AT RISK

An article with the title "Alcohol, or the search for a new kick" appeared in the medical daily *Le Généraliste* on 2 June 1996. It started with the words: "For some years, we have witnessed a massive increase in alcohol consumption among the young, whose sole aim is to get drunk." This is not just a French problem; it is to be found in many countries, particularly the United States, where over the last few years university campuses have been at the centre of a worrying increase in alcoholism.

A certain number of French surveys allow us to get an idea of the connection between teenagers and alcohol in general, and wine in particular.

Alcohol consumption of young people between the ages of 16 and 20 (1993)

Never drink	16%
Drink once a week	50%
Drink several times a week	28%
Drink every day	6%

(Source: CFES 1995)

When read in conjunction with other studies associated with this survey, this table of data shows a strong tendency among the majority of young people, to drink alcohol at the weekends and to get drunk with their friends. It is not a regular and moderate consumption. The frequency with which the young get drunk is quite revealing, as the following tables demonstrate:

Frequency of drunkenness among the young between the ages of 15 and 22 (1992)

Several times a term	5%
At least once a term	20%
Drunk at least once before the age of 16	33%

Young people drunk more than once a month (1993)

Sixth-formers	30%
Apprentices	18%
Military conscripts	31%

Age at which first drunk – data supplied by young people drunk at least 6 times a year (1994)

Between the ages of 12 and 13	5%
Between the ages of 14 and 15	18%
Between the ages of 16 and 17	33%
At the age of 18	49%

(Source: CFES 1995)

What is even more disturbing than the significant incidence of drunkenness among the young is the progression of this tendency over the last few years. In ten years, between 1978 and 1988, the incidence of repeated drunkenness among those between the ages of 15 and 19 went up threefold.

A particularly interesting conclusion arrived at by all the surveys, is that the young use beer and spirits to get drunk. One study, conducted in 1991, showed that young people in France drink two and a half times more beer than wine, and three and a half times more spirits, because they regarded drinking wine as "old fashioned".

Distribution of young people drinking wine between 1980 and 1995

Age Group	1980	1985	1990	1995
10-14	11.3%	4.3%	3.3%	2.0%
15-19	36.3%	18.0%	20.0%	18.8%

During the week they drink water and particularly drinks containing sugar (lemonades and colas), and at the weekend they get "stoned" on beer and particularly hard liquor. Quite recently a new generation of

183

alcoholic drinks targeting young people has emerged: Alco-pops. What effect these drinks will have on drunkenness among young people it is hard to say, but first signs give cause for concern.

Moreover, drinking fashions among the young reveal dangerous practices that are solely concerned with becoming drunk. Even in 1993, when a group of sixth-formers was asked why they drank alcohol, 52% said "for pleasure", 48% said "to help them forget" and 30% said they did it "to get drunk".

The serious questions we must therefore ask ourselves are: who and what is responsible for this sad situation, and what must be done to reverse the tendency.

THOSE RESPONSIBLE

The problem of alcoholism among the young must be seen as part of the problem of alcoholism in society as a whole, bearing in mind attitudes and policies that have developed over the course of recent years.

The brief and true story that follows is full of lessons that we ignore at our peril.

Simon is a 17-year-old boy who comes from a "good" middle-class family in Brittany. He has just gone into his final year at a private school where he is a boarder. He shares a room with Joseph, son of a small industrialist in the Bordeaux region. The boys get on well together and at Christmas Joseph invites his friend to spend a week with his family in their home near Arcachon.

Joseph's father has in his cellars some of the best wines from the Bordeaux region. At the same time, perhaps I should add that he prints and supplies labels to the majority of the best wine-producers in Bordeaux. Joseph's mother on the other hand, is a fantastic cook, as you so often find in those beautiful French provinces where gastronomy is still highly prized. In Joseph's family, wine is on the table at all meals, but it is always drunk in moderation. Knowing how to drink is part of the family's way of life: besides which, they never "drink" wine, they only "taste" it.

The children were initiated into wine tasting at an early age. When they were barely ten years old, their father began to help them discover, in homeopathic doses, the vintages and the varieties of grape not only from the prestigious vineyards of their region, but also from all the wine producing regions of France and the world. So much so, that at the age of 17, both Joseph and his sister one year his junior, could teach any wine waiter a thing or two.

It is a Sunday and as always, Joseph's father has brought up from his cellar some exceptional wines both to complete the education of his children and to honour Simon, the friend of his son.

As they have been served with a huge dish of Arcachon oysters, Joseph's father produces a bottle of white wine from an ice bucket that had been carefully hidden. "Children", he says mischievously looking at everyone, "I have here a first class vintage and I would like to know what you think of it!" And then, serving half a glass of the precious liquid to everyone at the table like a teacher who has just finished posing a problem, he declares: "I would like to know the region where the wine was produced, the grower, the grape variety and the year; and then I would like you to give me a pertinent description."

Already naturally shy, Simon froze. A feeling of panic started to overcome him when he saw each member of this strange family take their glass, make a few quick circular movements with it, thrust their noses into it and sniff, and then take several sips before declaring to the head of the family: "White Burgundy… Chablis… 1992… Chardonnay… straw colour… strong rich nose… with a hint of passion fruit… and a lingering finish…". "Good, good! Perfect! I am proud of you my children" said Joseph's father.

At that moment, the room suddenly went quiet. The whole family had just noticed that Simon had not touched his glass and sat rigidly in his seat like an Egyptian mummy.

"Well, Simon" said Joseph's father in surprise, "don't you like the Chablis?"

"I have never drunk wine, sir!", replied Simon.

"But at home, don't your parents drink a little wine?"

"No. When they go out, perhaps. But at home, we have never had wine. My mother is against alcohol. She says that there are already enough alcoholics in Brittany without adding to their numbers."

185

"How sad!" sighed Joseph's mother, with the same sorrowful air she would have used had Simon brought her some tragic news.

Two days later, Joseph was invited to the birthday of his cousin Sophie, who had asked him to bring Simon along as well. A few minutes after their arrival, the two friends were separated by the crowd, but a few hours later, when Joseph thought it was time to leave, he went out looking for his friend to take him home. He found him at the bar, totally drunk.

"Perhaps your friend has never drunk any wine in his life" ironically observed Sophie, "but he certainly knows all about whisky!"

During the rest of the academic year, Joseph noticed that each time Simon went out, he returned to school somewhat tipsy. So when Simon invited him to come and stay with him in Brittany, Joseph was rather curious to meet his water-drinking parents.

Simon's father is a judge, with a severe, angular face, who divides his time between the court and the loft at home, where he keeps his stamp collection. Simon's mother complements her husband: she is sad, always dressed in black, rather puritanical in appearance and slightly cantankerous. The family eats in the kitchen, dishes that have been prepared beforehand and then reheated in the microwave. As far as the mother is concerned, eating is a bit of a waste of time and alcoholism is her pet hate. She even belongs to a prohibitionist association.

During his stay, Joseph noticed that when the father emerged from his den in the loft, his eyes just that bit brighter than they had been before, he would start chewing a stick of liquorice even before he sat down to a meal. It suddenly dawned on Joseph, that the father of his friend was probably a secret drinker. A suspicion that was confirmed later by a friend of the family.

This story, which could have inspired Maupassant to write a novel, lays bare a regrettable situation for which the moral and particularly the political authorities in France are indirectly responsible. In any case, we can at least draw two conclusions with regard to the rules that should be adopted when talking about alcoholic drinks.

A negative, prohibitionist message stating baldly that "alcohol is dangerous and should be forbidden" merely incites people to break the rules and opens the door to alcohol abuse. On the other hand, a positive message stressing the cultural, gastronomic and medical perspectives associated with wine can lead to an easy, natural self-control.

To convince themselves, the public authorities need only look at the statistics and the distribution of alcoholism in France. It is, in fact, very striking to see that alcoholism in a region is inversely proportional to the importance of the wine industry there. Put in another way, the more wine produced in a region (like Bordeaux or Burgundy), the lower the incidence of alcoholism. The regions where alcoholism is at its highest are those regions where they produce no wine – like the North of France and Brittany.

The comparative index of male deaths due to cirrhosis of the liver – a frequent complication associated with alcoholism – in the period between 1988 and 1990, shows wide variations between one region of France and another. It is, in fact, much higher in the regions where they do not produce wine.

Based on an average figure of 100, details are as follows:

South-Pyrenees	58
Languedoc-Rousillon	66
Provence	73
South-West	76
Paris Area	83
Rhone-Alpes	90
Centre	123
Brittany	131
North – Calais Area	181

Robert Tinlot, Director General of the International Office for Vines and Wine, has told us:

"When I was head of the Agricultural College for the Manche et l'Ille-et-Vilaine (in the North of France), I had serious problems with alcoholism among my students. From the day that I was moved to Mâcon in Burgundy, all those problems disappeared."

This surely shows that information, education and an understanding about wine are the best weapons with which to fight alcohol abuse.

The survey conducted in the area of Bordeaux is particularly interesting from this point of view. It is the region with the lowest mortality rate due to alcoholic abuse in France: 28% below the national average. Life expectancy there is higher than the national average, since the incidence of illness and accidents is lower. The incidence of cardiovascular disease (particularly heart attacks), suicide, alcohol-related cancers and mental illness are substantially lower than the national average.

NEO-PROHIBITIONISM

From 1919 to 1933, the wind of Puritanism blew through the United States and into Scandinavia. Norway and Finland also introduced very strict measures to control the sale and consumption of alcohol. It was the era of Prohibition.

The result was a disaster. Firstly, because the mean consumption of alcohol increased considerably during this period, which was exactly the opposite of what was intended. And secondly, the production and sale of illicit alcohol controlled by the Mafia, generated a parallel economy which operated totally outside the law and gave rise to a bloody settling of accounts and a series of very sad scandals.

When dealing with alcohol, all governments should realise "it is forbidden to forbid". That is why any attempt to limit or reduce alcohol excess must be undertaken with the collaboration of all the professionals. Which is precisely what Mr Evin failed to do when he managed to get his law passed in 1991. It was a classic error of its type and achieved exactly the opposite of what was intended.

The authors of the Evin law, introduced during the socialist government of Michel Rocard, had as their objective the reduction of alcoholism in France and they thought that they would achieve this goal by introducing restrictive measures regarding the advertising of all alcoholic drinks.

This law, whose application orders still remained to be published in 1997, has been the object of intense controversy. Its detractors not only point out that it will not achieve what it sets out to do, but that it will also have a negative effect on important sectors of the economy, particularly in the world of advertising and in the media, and that it will bring about a massive reduction in sponsorship for sport.

In the text of this law, we find expressed all the prejudices of those involved in public hygiene and we can see that it is inspired, in fact, by the Ledermann law – a theoretical model used to analyse alcoholism based on the assumption that the causes are external to the individual, to his particular psychology and to his genetic characteristics. In other words, the problem lies with the product: alcohol.

It is not the objective of the Evin law that is criticised. Everybody is agreed that we should fight the curse of alcoholism. It is the means used which are in question. In attacking advertising, the Evin law is aiming at the wrong target. Ninety percent of the people who drink alcohol are moderate drinkers. The remaining ten percent drink to excess, drink irregularly or chronically. There is therefore no reason to impose restrictive measures on 90% of those drinkers that are moderate, particularly as the benefits of reasonable drinking have been amply demonstrated.

According to the government deputy Yves Rousset-Rouard, the reasons for the failure of this law are many and various:

"The authors of the Evin law wrongfully thought that a reduction in the level of publicity given to alcoholic drinks could lead to a reduction in the consumption of alcohol. However, this basic assumption is flawed for two main reasons. On the one hand, it has been accepted for some time that the principal effect of publicity is not to increase the general level of consumption but to strengthen the bond with those that consume the product. The publicity associated with alcoholic drinks is no exception to this rule. On the other hand, many scientific studies show that there is no link between the amount spent on advertising and the amount of alcohol consumed, and even less between the amount spent on advertising and the abuse of alcohol. In effect, it is shown both statistically and medically that alcohol abuse is a medical problem, independent of the amount of alcohol consumed by the market as a whole.

"Today, the failure of the Evin law is not even contested. Not only has it neither modified nor accelerated the general reduction in alcohol consumption in France over a period of fifteen years, experience shows that it has had no significant effect on alcohol abuse which, particularly with young people, has increased dramatically over the last few years."

In 1994, a survey conducted by the Institute IPSOS revealed that 75% of the French people thought that the attempt to limit advertising on alcoholic drinks as a way of fighting alcoholism was unlikely to be effective. In addition, 77% of those thought that the Evin law had little or no effect on the level of alcohol consumption. The decree that plans to allow poster advertising only in those areas where the alcoholic drinks are produced, was considered by the French to be absurd (67%), hypocritical (65%) and ineffective (85%).

For Thierrry Mantoux, the result of the study done by the organisation Enterprise and Prevention, of which he is the president, is quite unambiguous: "From this evaluation, it is clear that the benefits of the Evin law to public health are more than hypothetical, whereas the negative effects on the economy are more than obvious." On the question of public health, Enterprise and Prevention have noticed a drop in overall consumption by the young whilst at the same time there has been an increase in the incidence of drunkenness. This of course, contradicts the model underlying the Evin law, which predicts that alcohol abuse will decline with the reduction of overall consumption. At the economic level, the same organisation underlines two major disadvantages of the Evin law as far as producers of alcoholic drinks are concerned. Firstly, in order to strengthen the bond with the consumer, their investments have to be significantly higher than they were before the law was introduced, and this imposes a considerable burden. Secondly, the restrictive measures introduced by the law indirectly favour the sale of cheap products to the disadvantage of quality products, which cannot be explained and justified to the public. And yet, after 30 years, it has been because professionals have been able to use the media to put across their message to the public, that the quantity of wine consumed has been reduced in favour of promoting quality.

In 1988 and 1995, three studies conducted in the United States demonstrated there is no link between publicity and consumption. A study by

Professor Fisher came to the conclusion that publicity conducted in a mature market does not increase consumption but rather helps to diversify choice, to redistribute the market. As Jean-Guillaume d'Hérouville has said: "If Total and Elf conduct aggressive publicity campaigns, it will not cause people to travel further, rather they will come to prefer one brand of petrol to another."

But what is perhaps the most disquieting aspect of the Evin law, according to Alain-Gérard Slama, is the philosophy that goes with it. This stems from a puritanical tendency to "normalise morals or induce political correctness, where the State defines the behavioural norms of the whole population, establishing in this way a preventive order. However, the abuse of prevention, due to the fear of risk and conflict, ends by reducing the area of individual liberty and of depriving the citizen of his sense of responsibility, that is to say his means of liberty". However, as the government deputy Yves Rousset-Rouard has regretfully acknowledged: "the Evin law was adopted without any real co-ordination, without prior comparative analysis with other European countries and ignoring completely the contribution to the problem of alcoholism made by the individual."

In 1990, during the course of the World Cup in Italy, the whole world was able to read the advertisements for their wines proudly displayed at the various football stadia. In 1998, thanks to the Evin law, France will forbid the advertising of famous French wines on the grandstands at the St Denis Stadium. No doubt, in their stead will be the names of Coca Cola, Schweppes, Canada Dry – typical French products, as everyone knows!

THE ANTI-WINE CAMPAIGN

Since 15 September 1995, the maximum accepted level of alcohol in the blood for a driver in France has been set at 0.5g/l. It had been set less rigorously at 0.7g/l in July 1994 after having been at 0.8g/l for many years before that. But it was finally set at 0.5g/l in order to harmonise with regulations in Europe, and was accepted – according to the public authorities – "by a large consensus of the population" in France.

It is true that when you learn that nearly 40% of drivers involved in fatal road accidents are over the legal limit for alcohol in the blood, you are obliged to accept the logic behind the legislation. Although, as one taxi driver pointed out with all the common sense of his profession: "The day when the permitted alcohol level is reduced to 0.0001%, the authorities will be able to say that 99% of all fatal road accidents were caused by drivers over the legal limit." Adding with a certain amount of humour: "And when they need to show that they have the situation under control again, all they will have to do will be to legalise a higher level of alcohol in the blood."

But of course, when we come to plot the number of road accidents against the levels of alcohol in the blood of the drivers involved, we find that there is a real proportional increase in the risk factor when we go above 0.7g/l. Which is to say that if the level of alcohol in the blood is 1.2g/l, a driver has a three and a half times greater risk of having an accident that if he had no alcohol in his blood at all. If he has a level of 2g/l, the risk is multiplied by 80. Nobody can reasonably argue with legislation that is based on this sort of data, even if it is felt to be restrictive and repressive.

What we may legitimately quarrel with – even deplore – is the way the campaigns to encourage people to abide by the law can be conducted. In France, a bottle of red wine with glasses seems to be an ideal image to put before the public as the symbol of all that is bad in alcohol. In Holland recently, the authorities used posters featuring a Champagne bottle embodying all the sins associated with alcohol. We know of course, that this image is a perversion of the truth. The publicists acting for the government know it – at least, if they are properly informed, they should know it! – but the wider public does not, and it is inexcusable that professionals should use symbols for their own convenience, without having due regard to the unjustified damage they cause as a result.

But let us return to the question of fatal road accidents and the incontestable fact that 40% of the drivers involved in these accidents are over the legal limit. Some might reasonably believe that the people who cause these accidents are alcoholics. However, further investigation into the statistics can be very revealing.

The statistics are quite clear. In 85% of all fatal car accidents linked to alcohol, those responsible are occasional drinkers. Further, three-quarters of the accidents occur at night and mainly at the weekends, and they are

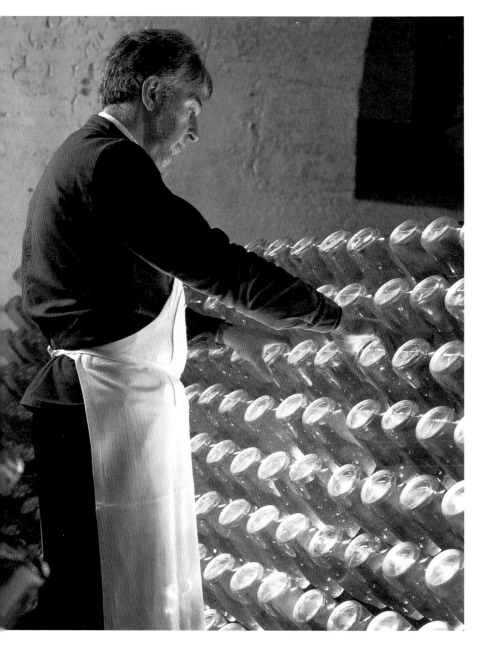

Performing the remuage on bottles of "Cristal" Champagne in the cellars of Louis Roederer.   *Reims, France.*

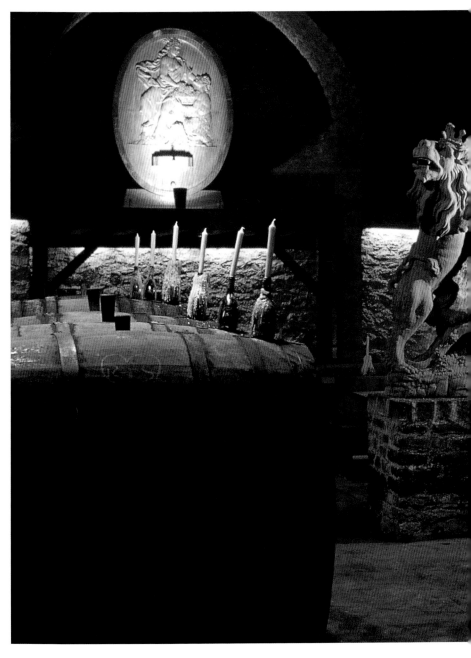

Würzburg Residenz wine cellar.   *Würzburg, Franken, Germany.*

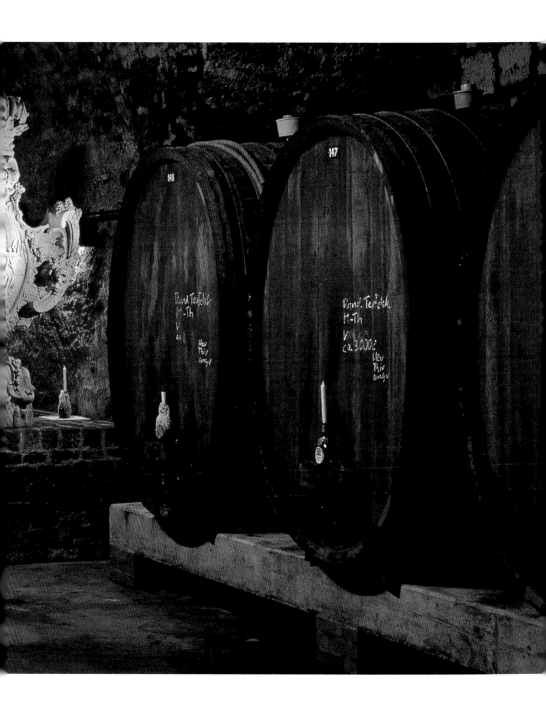

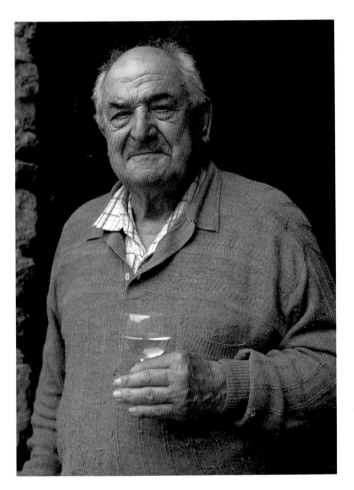

Alexis Guirouilh with a glass of his Jurançon moelleux.

caused by people (mainly young people) who only drink when they socialise at the end of the week. Usually they are people who do not drink during the week, but "let their hair down" at the weekends and are caught unawares by the effects of alcohol. Surprisingly, only rarely are alcoholics involved in these accidents (15%), since the regular nature of their drinking apparently makes them better able to cope with the effects alcohol.

What should be underlined is that regular, moderate drinkers practically never cause fatal car accidents in France within the terms that we have used during the course of this book. In fact, these moderate, regular drinkers are the sort of citizen the state should go out of its way to cultivate. First of all, because they rarely cause accidents. Secondly, because they normally drink wine (2 to 4 glasses a day on average) and therefore benefit from the health-giving properties it affords; which in turn, means they are less of a drain on the National Health Service and therefore save the State money. And thirdly, because they make a worthwhile contribution to the French economy and heritage, by maintaining the wine industry.

And of course it is precisely this category of responsible citizen that is reviled and persecuted by maladroit and misinformed anti-alcohol campaigns.

These anti-alcoholic campaigns have traumatised regular, moderate drinkers into becoming paranoid, like Simon's mother. By cultivating prohibitionist attitudes, all they have succeeded in doing is throw oil on the fire and indirectly encouraging alcoholism, particularly among the young.

HELPING PEOPLE TO DRINK WISELY

It is April 1996. We are in the sixth form of a small town school in the Rhône-Alpes region of France, at the centre of one of the most prestigious wine growing areas of the Rhône valley. As he does each year, the biology teacher has taken his final year students on a trip to the important wine cellars belonging to the local co-operative.

Because the students will have to write a report on the visit, trained guides ply them with lots of details regarding the different stages in the preparation of wine. After a scintillating talk by a great oenologist, the class is invited to have a light snack before going back to school. Imagine the amazement of the pupils when they assemble in the dining room, to find that the only refreshment on offer is lemonade and Coca Cola!

To calm down the noisy and offended students, the teacher decided to make them aware of the situation. "I think you ought to know" he said, "that I had to fight tooth and nail to get permission for you to come here today. I succeeded, but only on condition that you should not be given any wine to drink, at all."

The situation is totally farcical. Here we have a group of 35 young people, between the ages of 17 and 19, being offered an intelligent introduction to wine and its traditions, and they are not even allowed to taste it. With reactionary attitudes like this in education, it is small wonder we have a problem with alcoholism among the young!

Fortunately, it is more than likely that all these young people had already served their cultural apprenticeship at home, where they had been taught how to drink wisely. After all, eight of them come from families owning vineyards. However, the intolerance, hypocrisy and stupidity displayed by the educational authorities in this case beggars belief. What were these people afraid of? That one of the parents would hold them responsible before the Ministry of Education for inciting their offspring to become an alcoholic?

So long as objective information is not properly organised and made readily available to the public, aberrations like the one just examined will continue to exist. For we are currently in a Manichean situation, where two "religions" are in direct confrontation: the neo-prohibitionists on the one side and the advocates of drinking with moderation on the other. But the battle is not fairly balanced because the latter are being strangled by the clichés of political expediency. Bearing this in mind, it is clearly a matter of great urgency that those advocating moderation evolve a radically new way of communicating with the world.

Wine growing experts, teachers, doctors and public authorities must combine to ensure that they are always objective and open-minded. However, it is primarily at family level that teaching the world to drink wisely should begin.

DRINKING WISELY WITHIN THE FAMILY

In his book *Eating differently*, Professor Joyeux, the father of a large family, said that learning how to appreciate and drink wine should start when a child is ten years old. And he was right. Children should be initiated quite early into the mysteries of wine, so that it can become fully integrated into their background and way of life. This is why wine should be a familiar sight in the home, drunk in a regular and moderate way.

Children should also be made aware that wine is not a drink to quench their thirst. Water is far more suitable for that purpose. Rather, wine is a food that should be tasted.

Very early on, children should begin to sense the mystery surrounding wine, begin to know how it is made and be allowed to discover the variety of vintages and qualities. At lunch on Sunday or at dinner parties, when dishes are normally more elaborate and sophisticated, they should be given the opportunity to help select a finer wine more suited to the occasion. Even if their parents live in an apartment, it is normally possible to find a corner that is cooler or darker than the rest, where a modest cellar can be assembled. Ideally, it may be possible to acquire a room below ground that is not heated or perhaps buy a temperature controlled wine cupboard.

It is very important that children should see that wine is treated with care and allowed to rest, even if only for a short while. It is essential too, that they should not see it pass straight from the shopping bag onto the meal table, because this would tend to give it the character of a commodity and remove its mystery.

Parents happening to live in a wine growing area, should take their children to see the wine harvest and visit the cellars where the wine is stored and, whenever possible, explore the complex culture associated with wine. In this way, the mystery of wine will become a living experience devoid of taboos and children will grow into adulthood at ease with wine, as with a good friend. And when all is said and done, which one among us will abuse a good friend?

One thing is for sure. Excluding all alcoholic drink from the family table is probably the best way of raising it to "forbidden fruit" status. And we all know of course what happened in the Garden of Eden!

It is an approach that can easily be applied outside the home, particularly at school. It is also an approach that could well inform the actions and statements of those who operate in the public domain.

The campaign "Thirst to Live", conducted in Nancy and in Le Havre in 1993, was very interesting in terms of informing teenagers about the risks associated with drinking in specific situations, at discos, in groups and on the road. It targeted teenagers between the ages of 16 and 20, but it should have included younger people as well. However, the organisers had the good sense to avoid moralising, as this would have been totally counter-productive.

This kind of initiative deserves to be mentioned, but it must be admitted that it only limits the damage likely to affect those most at risk. It does not solve the real problem, which requires working with children at a much younger age.

This awareness underlay the suggestion of Dr Pierre Bébéar at the European Parliament that his colleagues should adopt the principle of introducing wine education into school curricula. Were this to happen, it would be a real revolution in the educational field; but there is some way to go yet before deep-seated attitudes and taboos finally disappear.

CONCLUSION

For many years, Morley Safer had been one of the big stars of American television with his Sunday evening programme *Sixty Minutes* on CBS Network. However, his reputation increased enormously after he had the courage to broadcast two programmes on the theme of "Wine and Health". One of these programmes was broadcast in 1991 on *The French Paradox*. The other was broadcast in 1995 on *The Danish Study*, which is included in Appendix 1.

In a country where there are powerful anti-alcohol lobbies and the spectre of Prohibition is always present in the collective unconscious, it required considerable courage to pronounce on television that a drink containing alcohol could be good for your health.

What is even more surprising, is that barely two months after this scoop, the American authorities incorporated the new findings in their official dietary advice bulletin. In this they said that a moderate and regular consumption of wine could, for certain individuals, be associated with a reduced risk of coronary disease.

However, these new recommendations by the Americans are expressed with considerable caution with regard to the amounts of wine that are admissible: 15 cl per day for women and 30 cl for men.

And yet this is already higher that the average level of consumption in France, which has now fallen to 20 cl per adult per day.

Here we have good cause to reflect upon the mysteries associated with preconceived ideas.

APPENDIX 1

THE DANISH STUDY

Authors: Gronbaek M, Deis A, Sorensen T I A, Becker U, Schnohr P, Jensen G

Source: British Medical Journal, vol.310 – 6 May 1995

Title: *Mortality associated with moderate intakes of wine, beer or spirits*

SUMMARY

Design: Population study with baseline assessment of alcohol intake, smoking habit, income, education and body mass index, with 10-12 year follow up of mortality.

Setting: Copenhagen City, heart study.

Subjects: 6,051 men and 7,234 women aged 30 – 70 years.

Main outcome measure:
Number and time of cause-specific deaths from 1976 to 1988.

Results: The risk of dying steadily decreased with an increasing intake of wine – from a relative risk of 1.00 for the subjects who never drank wine to 0.51 (95% confidence interval 0.32 to 0.81) for those who drank three to five glasses a day. However, intake of neither beer nor spirits was associated with a reduced risk. For spirits intake, the relative risk of dying increased from 1.00 for those who never drank, to 1.34 (1.05 to 1.71) for those with an intake of three to five drinks a day. The effects of the three types of alcoholic drinks seemed to be independent of each other, and no significant interactions existed with sex, age, education, income, smoking or body mass index. Wine drinking showed the same relation to risk of death from cardio-vascular disease as to risk of death from all causes.

Conclusion: Low to moderate intake of wine is associated with lower mortality from cardiovascular and cerebrovascular disease

and other causes. Similar intake of spirits implied an
increased risk, while beer drinking did not affect mortality.

INTRODUCTION

During the past decade, several large population studies have shown a
U-shaped relation between alcohol intake and mortality for both men
and women throughout adulthood. (1)(2)(3)(4)(5)(6)

In a recent study we found that the U shape persisted when the effects
of other risk factors, such as smoking and obesity, were controlled. (7)

Furthermore, neither a higher prevalence of disease at baseline nor
an increased number of former drinkers among non-drinkers can explain
the U shape. (7)(8)

The risk function for all cause mortality may be the result of combined
effects of a decreasing risk of coronary heart disease and an increasing
risk of cirrhosis, cancers, and violent deaths, due to an increasing intake.
(4)

St Leger and colleagues (9) and more recently Renaud and colleagues
(10) found an inverse relation between incidence of coronary heart
disease and wine consumption in different countries but no such relation
for beer consumption. This suggests that the type of alcoholic drink, in
addition to alcohol itself, influences the risk of heart disease. Some
studies have addressed the issue of type of drink and death from heart
disease but did so rather superficially and gave conflicting results.
(11)(12)(13)(14)(15)(16)(17)

In a recent paper specifically addressing this question, Klatsky and
Armstrong suggested that people who drink wine may be better protected
against death from coronary heart disease than those who drink other
alcoholic beverages, but proper risk functions were not estimated. (18)

We assess the effects of different types of alcoholic drinks on the risk
of death from all causes and from cardiovascular and cerebrovascular
disease, while taking into account, sex, age, socio-economic conditions,
smoking habits and body mass index.

SUBJECTS AND METHODS

Population

The study population comprised a random, age stratified sample of 19,698 of 87,172 individuals aged 20 or more, living in the Osterbro area of Copenhagen in 1976. During 1976-8, the Copenhagen City heart study, examined by questionnaire 14,223 subjects (6,511 men, 7,712 women; response rate 72.2%). A detailed description of the study procedure has been published previously.(19) The present analysis concerns a sample of 13,285 subjects (6,051 men, 7,234 women) aged 30 – 79.

Examination procedures

The subjects filled in a self-administered questionnaire about various issues related to health, including alcohol intake, smoking habits, school education and household income. Weight in light clothes and height without shoes were measured, and from these the body mass index (weight(kg)/height((m).sup.2)) was calculated.

Alcohol intake – The subjects were asked in multiple choice form, whether they drank beer (bottles), wine (glasses) or spirits (units) "hardly ever/never", "monthly", "weekly" or "daily". If a subject drank alcohol daily, then he or she had to report the average number of drinks of each type taken each day. One bottle of beer contains 12g of alcohol, and this may be considered the average for the other types of drinks. If a subject abstained from drinking alcohol because he or she was receiving treatment (for example, disulfiram) or because of dipsomania, then this was noted, and the subject was excluded from the analysis.

Smoking habits – The subjects reported if they had never smoked, were former smokers or current smokers. Former smokers were divided into groups according to duration (in years) of non-smoking and current smokers, according to amount of tobacco (in grams smoked each day). For the analysis, five groups were defined: subjects who had never smoked; former smokers who had not smoked for more than five years; former smokers who had not smoked for five years or less; smokers of 1-19g tobacco daily; smokers of more than 19g daily.

Follow up

We followed the survival of the population sample until 1 January 1988, using the unique person identification number in the national central person register. We obtained causes of death, as recorded on death certificates, from the National Board of Health. Death from cardio-vascular and cerebrovascular disease was defined according to the International Classification of Diseases, eighth revision, as codes 410.0 to 445.9. Each subject was observed from their initial examination (1976-8) until 1st January 1988, or until death (2,229), disappearance (one) or emigration (39) if these occurred earlier.

Statistical analysis

Data was analysed with multiple Poisson regression models. (20) The mortality was assumed to be constant within each 10 year age interval. A subject who was observed in more than one age group, contributed with corresponding observation time in both groups. Further details of the model analysis have been described previously. (7)

The model included the subjects' age, sex and intakes of beer, wine and spirits, and the first order interactions between these variables. Each type of alcoholic drink was classified as never drunk; drunk monthly; drunk weekly; one or two drinks a day; or three to five drinks a day. Subjects having more than five drinks a day of beer, wine or spirits were excluded from this analysis because there were too few cases in some of the groups (see table 1). Exclusion of subjects who had more than five drinks a day of one type of alcoholic drink meant that some subjects who had less than five drinks daily of the other types were excluded. In this model first order interactions were tested. The criterion for inclusion was significance at the 5% level. We added the following covarieties to this reduced model: smoking, body mass index, school education and income. These were added one by one for separate testing.

TABLE 1 – Distribution of alcohol intake and number of deaths from all causes and from cardiovascular and cerebrovascular disease in 13,285 subjects aged 30 – 79 years, by sex and type of alcoholic drink.

MEN

Alcoholic drink	Total number of persons	Total number of deaths	Deaths from cardio-vascular and cerebrovascular disease
BEER			
Never	987	286	164
Monthly	1123	221	138
Weekly	1521	293	165
Daily: 1-2 drinks	1126	288	161
3-5 drinks	881	200	90
< 6 drinks	413	110	47
WINE			
Never	2553	780	421
Monthly	2304	433	241
Weekly	930	134	72
Daily: 1-2 drinks	195	42	24
3-5 drinks	62	8	6
< 6 drinks	7	1	1
SPIRITS			
Never	2305	617	336
Monthly	2241	388	216
Weekly	992	219	120
Daily: 1-2 drinks	361	118	65
3-5 drinks	152	56	28
< 6 drinks	0	0	0
TOTALS	6051	1398	765

WOMEN

Alcoholic drink	Total number of persons	Total number of deaths	Deaths from cardio-vascular and cerebrovascular disease
BEER			
Never	3738	499	228
Monthly	1931	161	61
Weekly	1123	114	41
Daily: 1-2 drinks	378	50	21
3-5 drinks	54	6	3
< 6 drinks	10	1	0
WINE			
Never	3037	473	234
Monthly	2820	251	91
Weekly	1046	84	21
Daily: 1-2 drinks	256	19	7
3-5 drinks	68	4	1
< 6 drinks	7	0	0
SPIRITS			
Never	4062	523	229
Monthly	2193	198	76
Weekly	688	66	23
Daily: 1-2 drinks	254	40	25
3-5 drinks	37	4	1
< 6 drinks	0	0	0
TOTALS	7234	831	354

In another model, the risk of dying as a function of reported intake at baseline, was estimated separately for the first six years and the second six years. For detailed description of the statistical methods, we refer to the recently published statistical appendix. (7)

RESULTS

Table 1 shows the distribution of subjects according to the different types of alcoholic drink. Some subjects who never drank alcohol of one type, drank one or two of the others. Thus 1,116 subjects never drank beer but did drink wine or spirits, 1,245 never drank wine but did drink beer or spirits, and 860 never drank spirits but did drink beer or wine. In all, 5,858 subjects drank both wine and beer, 5,408 drank both spirits and wine, and 4,629 drank both spirits and beer. Only 77 subjects drank wine, beer and spirits every day. A total of 2,120 women and 625 men never drank any alcohol.

During follow-up, 831 women and 1,398 men died; 354 of the women and 765 of the men died from cardiovascular or cerebrovascular disease. The number of deaths analysed was reduced by 275, owing to exclusion of subjects who had more than five drinks of one type of alcohol. In the models for all cause mortality and mortality from cardiovascular or cerebrovascular disease including age, sex, smoking and intake of beer, wine or spirits, all first order interactions (except interaction between age and sex) were not significant. Thus intake of beer, wine or spirits appeared independently associated with mortality in this population. Estimates are reported from the models including all three types of alcoholic drinks.

Smoking was a confounder as the subjects who drank any type of alcoholic drink were more likely to smoke than those who did not drink at all, and where smoking influenced mortality. The reported results are therefore controlled for smoking. We found no significant effect however, of education, income, or body mass index on the relation between any of the types of drink and mortality.

Wine intake and mortality

The wine drinkers experienced a significantly lower all cause mortality than the subjects who drank no wine. When relative risk was set at 1.00 for subjects who never drank wine the risk steadily decreased to 0.51 (95% confidence interval 0.32 to 0.81) for subjects who drank three to five glasses of wine a day (figure). The risk of death from cardiovascular and cerebrovascular disease declined from 1.00 for non-drinkers to 0.4 (0.24

to 0.80) for drinkers of three to five glasses of wine a day (Table 2). With regard to causes of death other than cardiovascular and cerebrovascular disease, drinking wine implied a decreased risk compared with not drinking wine (Table 2).

TABLE 2 – Relative risk (95% confidence interval) of death related to coronary disease and other causes, as a function of alcoholic drink consumption for 13,285 people aged between 30 and 79 years.

Frequency	Beer consumption	Wine consumption	Spirit consumption
Death due to cardiovascular disease and cerebrovascular disease			
Never (reference)	1.00	1.00	1.00
Monthly	0.79 (0.69-0.91)	0.69 (0.62-0.77)	0,95 (0.85-1.06)
Weekly	0.87 (0.79-0.99)	0.53 (0.45-0.63)	1.08 (0.93-1.26)
Daily: 1-2 drinks	0.79 (0.68-0.91)	0.47 (0.35-0.62)	1.16 (0.98-1.39)
3-5 drinks	0.72 (0.61-0.88)	0.44 (0.24-0.80)	1.35 (1.00-1.83)
Death due to other causes			
Never (reference)	1.00	1.00	1.00
Monthly	0.82 (0.71-0.95)	0.86 (0.77-0.97)	0.80 (0.71-0.91)
Weekly	1.02 (0.89-1.18)	0.86 (0.64-0.88)	0.92 (0.79-1.08)
Daily: 1-2 drinks	0.96 (0.84-1.15)	0.80 (0.62-1.03)	0.81 (0.65-0.99)
3-5 drinks	1.22 (1.02-1.45)	0.50 (0.27-0.91)	1.36 (1.01-1.84)

Beer intake and mortality

We found no trend in all cause mortality in relation to the subjects who drank beer daily, compared with the subjects who never drank beer, but we found a slight, significant decrease in risk among those who drank beer monthly. The relative risk was 0.96 (0.86 to 1.07) for subjects who drank beer weekly and 0.95 (0.83 to 1.09) for those who drank three to five beers a day. With respect to death from cardiovascular and cerebrovascular disease, intake of three to five beers a day implied a reduction risk of 0.72 (0.61 to 0.88) compared with not drinking beer (Table 2).

Spirits intake and mortality

As with wine and beer, monthly intake of spirits was associated with a slight, significant decrease in risk, but drinking spirits weekly or once or twice a day, did not influence all cause mortality compared with not drinking spirits at all. An intake of three to five drinks a day however, was associated with a significantly increased risk of 1.34 (1.05 to 1.71) compared with not drinking spirits. The risk function between intake of spirits and mortality from cardiovascular and cerebrovascular disease showed the same pattern as the one for all cause mortality (Table 2).

Stability of risk functions

The analysis was repeated with the observation time divided into the first and second six-year periods. The increased mortality among subjects who did not drink wine compared with those who drank wine daily, persisted in the second period.

DISCUSSION

We clearly distinguished the different types of alcoholic drinks with respect to their relation to all cause mortality and mortality from cardio-vascular and cerebrovascular disease. We found that the descending part of the U-shaped curve describing the relation between alcohol and mortality could be explained almost exclusively be the effect of drinking wine. Furthermore, our study showed that the first part of the ascending curve (the increasing mortality among heavy drinkers) may be explained primarily by the effect of drinking spirits.

Validity of reported intake

The validity of self-reported alcohol intake may be questioned, but no other available methods (such as sales reports, collateral information) have proved to be more valid. (21) We have no reason to believe that

211

drinkers of one type of alcoholic drink, report their intake differently from drinkers of other types. If underreporting takes place, as is commonly assumed, then this would lower the estimated health damaging effect of spirits, moving the "true" threshold of hazardous drinking to the right. On the other hand, the estimated beneficial effect of wine, if it were related to an even greater intake, would appear even more striking. Thus if underreporting takes place, the estimated beneficial effect of say three to five glasses of wine a day, would relate to a greater intake. The results may therefore be considered conservative estimates of the true differences in the effects of the different drinks.

We found no excess mortality among subjects who did not drink beer or spirits. Of course, the presence of sick non-drinkers could mask a possible beneficial effect of not drinking beer or spirits. For wine drinking, the presence of sick no-drinkers would contribute to the inverse risk function. We also analysed however, the mortality risk function in the first and second six years of follow-up and found no changes between the two periods. Furthermore, only a fraction of non-drinkers of one of the three types of drink were also non-drinkers of the other two types. Sick non-drinkers are probably not, therefore, imposing an important bias on the results.

Analyses of effects of type of alcoholic drinks

The descending part of the U shaped curve describing the relation between alcohol and mortality has been attributed to a protective effect of ethanol, but the question of type of alcoholic drink has been addressed rather superficially. Some studies have mentioned having controlled for, or by other means included, the type of drink in the analysis – with little or no difference in effect on mortality. (11)(12)(13)(14)(15)(16) Others have addressed the question specifically, but may have had too small a material or too little variance in intake of the different drinks to detect differences. (1)(17)(22) An ecological study reported that it is apparently an advantage, with respect to coronary heart disease, to live in a country of wine drinkers rather than in a country of drinkers of beer or spirits. (10) This finding was supported by Klatsky and Armstrong, who indicated that people who preferred wine may have a lower risk of dying from coronary heart disease. (18) Klatsky and Armstrong grouped subjects according to preference of a given type of drink. This might have led to loss of information as well as misclassification because many subjects presumably drank two or all three types of drink. Klatsky and Armstrong's method of classification might also have hindered comparison between drinkers of different types of drinks and the group of non-drinkers of each type of drink.

An important difference between the studies mentioned above and our study is that we specifically addressed not only the question of separate effects of the different types of alcoholic drinks on mortality, but also the question of possible interactions between the types of alcoholic drinks on mortality. A remarkable methodological advantage in conducting the study in Denmark, is that the Danes – in contrast with people in countries with a more uniform pattern of drinking or a culture of non-drinking – drink some of all type of alcoholic drink, which enabled us to create the five intake groups for wine, beer and spirits. Drinking one type of alcohol will affect the pattern of drinking another. The statistical model should therefore include all three types of alcohol. We found no significant interaction between the three types of alcoholic drinks and could therefore provide estimates of independent effect of each type (ranging from never drinking to having three to five drinks daily of that type) on mortality.

The left side of the U-shaped curve has been the subject of much debate. A prevailing belief is that the non-drinkers constitute a mixture of former heavy drinkers, drinkers who underreport, sick people who have stopped drinking, and people with a particularly unhealthy lifestyle apart from not drinking. As seen in Table 1 for each of the three types of drink, quite a large group of subjects were non-drinkers. Patients taking disulfiram and patients with dipsomania were excluded from that analysis. The influence of type of drink on mortality seemed to show that the drinks were statistically independent of each other, and the difference persisted throughout the 12 years of follow-up. Smoking is known to confound the estimates of the effect of alcohol intake on mortality, (7) and we therefore controlled for this factor. We found that wine intake was positively correlated with social class variables (data not shown), but the protective effect of wine, with regard to mortality, was not significantly weakened when we controlled for this factor. Sex, age, and body mass index did not confound our results either. Residual

213

confounding by some of the included variables or by other, unknown, confounders may none-the-less have occurred. To explain the effect however, such confounders would have to exhibit a peculiar distribution across the range of intakes of the three types of drinks. If a variable, such as physical activity, were a confounder (assuming that physical activity reduces mortality), then there should be an increase in physical activity by increased wine intake, decreased activity by increased spirits intake, and no change in relation to beer. Moreover, the effect of any such potential confounder should be very strong to explain our findings.

Possible protective factors in wine apart from Ethanol

The results strongly suggest that, in addition to the common effect of ethanol, there are – within the studied range of drinking – different factors influencing health in the three types of drink. Specifically, the results raise the question of what might be the protective agent in wine or the damaging factors in beer and spirits apart from ethanol. The decreased mortality in cardiovascular and cerebrovascular disease among beer drinkers may reflect a common effect of ethanol on high-density lipoprotein or fibrinolytic factors. (23) Furthermore, and inverse relation has been found between alcohol intake and platelet agreeability, (24) and – in agreement with our results – this relation has been shown to be even stronger for wine. (25) Our finding, that only wine drinking clearly reduces both the risk of dying from cardiovascular and cerebrovascular disease and the risk of dying from other causes, suggest that other more broadly acting factors in wine may be present. Antioxidants and flavonoids, which are presumed to prevent both coronary heart disease and some cancers, (26)(27) may be present in red wine. It has also been suggested that tannin and other phenolic compounds in red wine, may have a protective effect. (28)(29)

The number of drinks indicating the lowest risk on the alcohol-mortality risk function, as well as the thresholds of safe drinking, differs from study to study, and this variation may be due to differences between countries with regard to type of drinks consumed.

During the past 15 years, mortality from coronary heart disease has declined by about 30% in Denmark. (30) This decrease cannot be ascribed to arise in alcohol intake, which has been more or less stable during that period. On the other hand, with the opening of the European market, drinking patterns have changed quite dramatically in favour of wine drinking. In 1975, wine contributed to 17.3% of the total alcohol intake, rising to 30.2% in 1922, (31) which – in accordance with our findings – may have contributed to the decline in death from coronary heart disease.

In conclusion, our study shows that light and moderate wine drinking, in contrast with beer and spirits drinking, is associated with a strong dose-dependent decrease in all cause mortality, attributable to a decrease in mortality from cardiovascular and cerebrovascular disease as well as from other causes.

The biological mechanism behind the different effects of the three types of drinks needs further research.

(1)   Kozararevic D, McGee D, Vojvodic N, Racic Z, Dawber T, Gordon T, et al. *Frequency of alcohol consumption and morbidity and mortality.* Lancet 1980; i:613-6

(2)   Marmot MG, Rose G, Shipley MJ, Thomas BJ. *Alcohol and mortality: a U-shaped curve.* Lancet 1981; I:580-3

(3)   Shaper AG, Wannamathee G, Walker M. *Alcohol and mortality in British men: explaining the U-shaped curve.* Lancet 1988; i:1267-73

(4)   Bofetta P, Garfinkel L. *Alcohol drinking and mortality among men enrolled n an American Cancer Society prospective study.* Epidemiology 1990; 1:337-9.

(5)   Klatsky AL, Armstrong MA, Friedman GD. *Alcohol and mortality.* Ann Intern Med 1992; 117:646-54

(6)   Doll R, Peto R, Hall E, Wheatley K, Gray R. *Mortality in relation to consumption of alcohol: 13 years' observations on male British doctors.* BMJ 1994; 309:911-8

(7)   Gronhaek M, Deis A, Sorensen TIA, Becker U, Borch-Johnsen K, Muller C, et al. *Influence of age, gender, body mass index and smoking on alcohol intake and mortality.* BMJ 1994; 308:302-6

(8)   Jackson R, Scragg R, Beaglehole R. *Alcohol consumption and risk of coronary heart disease* BMJ 1991; 303:211-6

(9)   St Leger AS, Cochrane AL, Moore F. *Factors associated with cardiac mortality in developed countries with particular reference to the consumption of wine.* Lancet 1979; i:1017-20

(10) Renaud S, de Logeril M. *wine, alcohol, platelets and the French Paradox for coronary heart disease.* Lancet 1992; 339:1523-6

(11) Yano K, Rhoads GG, Kagan A. *Coffee, alcohol and risk of coronary heart disease among Japanese men living in Hawaii.* N Engl J Med 1977; 297;405-9

(12) Hennekens CH, Willet W, Rosner B, Cole DS, Myrent SL. *Effects of beer, wine and liquor on coronary deaths.* JAMA 1979; 242:1973-4

(13) Rosenberg L, Slone D, Shapirto S, Kaufman DW, Miettinen OS, Stolley PD. *Alcoholic beverages and myocardial infarction in young women.* Am J Public Health 1981; 71:82-5

(14) Klatsky AL, Armstrong MA,Friedman GD. *Relation of alcoholic beverage use to subsequent coronary heart disease hospitalisation.* Am J Cardiol 1986; 58:710-4

(15) Friedman LA, Kimball AW. *Coronary heart disease mortality and alcohol consumption in Framingham.* Am J Cardiol 1986; 124(3): 481-9

(16) Stampfer MJ, Colditz GC, Willet WC Spiezer FE, Hennekens CH. *A prospective study of moderate alcohol consumption and the risk of coronary heart disease and stroke in women.* N Engl J Med 1988; 319; 267-73

(17) Rimm EB, Giovannucci EL, Willett WC, Colditz GA, Ascherio A, Rosner B, et al. *Prospective study of alcohol consumption and risk of coronary disease in men.* Lancet 1991; 338:464-8

(18) Klatsky AL, Armstrong MA. *Alcoholic beverage choice and risk of coronary heart disease mortality: do red wine drinkers fare best?* Am J Cardiol 1993; 71:467-9

(19) Appleyard M, Hansen AT, Schnoh P, Jensen G, Nyboe. *The Copenhagen City heart study. A book of tables with data from the first examination (1976-78) and five year follow-up (1981-83).* J Soc Med 1989; 170 (supl.41): 1-160.

(20) McCullagh P, Nelder JA. *Generalised linear models.* New York: Chapman and Hall, 1983.

(21) Midanik L. *Validity of self-reported alcohol use: a literature review and assessment.* British Journal of Addiction 1988; 83:1019-29

(22) Kimball AW, Friedman LA, Moore RD. *Non-linear modelling of alcohol consumption for analysis of beverage type effect and beverage preference effect.* Am J Epidemiol 1992; 135:1287-92

(23) Hendricks HFJ, Veenstra J, Wiercik EJMV, Schaafsma G, Kluft C. *Effect of moderate dose of alcohol with evening meal on fibrinolytic factors.* BMJ 1994; 85:854-7

(24) Criqui MH. *The reduction of coronary heart disease with light to moderate alcohol consumption: effect of artificial?* British Journal of Addiction 1990; 85:854-7

(25) Seigneur M, Bonnet J, Dorian B, Benchimol D, Druouillet F, Gouverneur G, et al. *Effect of the consumption of alcohol, wine and red wine, on platelet function and serum lipids.* Journal of Applied Cardiology 1990; 5:215-22

(26) Hertog MG, Feskens EJ, Hollman PC, Katan MB, Kromhout D. *Dietary antioxidant flavonoids and risk of coronary heart disease: The Zutphen elderly study.* Lancet 1993; 342:1007-11

(27) Chen J, Geissler C, Parpia B, Li J, Campbell TC. *Antioxidant status and cancer mortality in China.* Int. J Epideiol 1992; 2:625-35

(28) Frankel EN, Kanner J, German JB, Parks E, Kinsella JE. *Inhibition of oxidation of human low-density lipoprotein by phenolic substances in red wine.* Lancet 1993; 341:454-7

(29) Carnacini A, Arfelli G. *Selected nutritional components of wine.* Alcologia 1994; 6:41-9

(30) Gerdes L. *A marked decline in the mortality of ischemic heart disease in middle-aged Danish men in the 1980's and simultaneous changes in the mortality from other causes.* Ugeskr Lager 1992; 154:3580-6

(31) Saelan H, Sindballe A-M, Schmidt D. *Alcohol and drug abuse 1992.* 21st ed. Copenhagen: National Board of Health, 1993

APPENDIX 2

Table 1

Analysis of alcohol consumption in 13 countries since 1961, compared to France (expressed in litres)

	Spirits	Beer	Wine	Pure alcohol Total in litres
FRANCE				
1961	2.17	37.2	126.1	17.7
1970	2.30	41.2	109.1	16.2
1980	2.50	44.3	91.0	14.9
1990	2.49	41.5	72.7	12.6
1994	2.49	40.0	63.0	11.4
UNITED KINGDOM				
1961	0.80-	89.2	1.82	4.5
1970	0.94	103.0	2.89	5.3
1980	1.78	118.3	7.19	7.3
1990	1.71	109.5	11.56	7.6
1994	1.56	102.3	12.65	7.5
UNITED STATES				
1961	2.08	56.9	3.55	5.1
1970	2.87	70.0	4.97	6.7
1980	3.07	92.0	7.87	8.2
1990	2.29	90.8	7.69	7.4
1994	1.96	85.2	6.00	6.6
BELGIUM				
1961	0.72	115.4	8.6	6.5
1970	1.32	132.4	14.2	8.9
1980	2.37	131.3	20.6	10.2
1990	1.20	120.7	24.9	9.9
1994	1.20	101.6	24.0	9.0

GERMANY

1961	2.12	101.6	12.2	7.4
1970	3.01	141.1	16.0	10.3
1980	3.05	145.7	15.5	11.4
1990	2.33	143.1	25.1	10.6
1994	2.40	139.6	22.6	10.3

GREECE

1961	–	5.3	41.9	5.3
1970	–	9.4	40.0	5.3
1980	3.5	26.3	44.9	10.2
1990	2.7	39.8	32.8	8.6
1994	2.7	42.0	33.8	8.9

ITALY

1961	1.2	6.1	108.2	12.3
1970	1.8	11.3	113.7	13.7
1980	1.9	16.7	92.9	13.0
1990	1.0	25.1	62.5	9.2
1994	0.9	26.2	58.5	8.7

JAPAN

1961	–	12.9	–	0.5
1970	1.07	28.1	0.32	4.6
1980	1.83	37.5	0.55	5.4
1990	2.2	52.3	1.09	6.5
1994	2.0	57.3	1.10	6.6

LUXEMBURG

1961	1.12	118.6	32.7	8.6
1970	1.73	127.0	37.0	10.0
1980	1.69	114.4	48.2	10.9
1990	1.57	121.4	58.2	12.2
1994	1.60	122.9	60.5	12.5

HOLLAND

1961	1.19	26.4	2.34	2.8
1970	2.09	57.4	5.15	5.7
1980	2.72	86.3	12.85	8.9
1990	1.98	87.7	14.54	8.1
1994	1.77	86.6	14.54	7.9

PORTUGAL

1961	–	4.9	99.3	12.2
1970	0.5	13.3	72.5	9.9
1980	0.9	37.9	68.7	11.0
1990	0.8	65.1	50.0	10.1
1994	0.8	77.1	50.7	10.7

SPAIN

1961	–	13.3	52.5	7.0
1970	2.3	38.5	61.5	11.6
1980	3.2	53.4	64.7	13.6
1990	2.7	71.9	37.4	10.8
1994	2.5	66.2	32.2	9.7

SWEDEN

1961	2.46	36.8	3.58	4.1
1970	2.64	57.5	6.37	5.8
1980	2.74	47.2	9.54	5.7
1990	1.72	59.8	12.24	5.5
1994	1.50	64.2	12.6	5.3

SWITZERLAND

1961	1.58	68.5	36.7	9.6
1970	1.94	70.5	41.9	10.7
1980	2.05	69.5	47.5	10.8
1990	1.78	69.8	49.4	10.8
1994	1.55	64.3	44.3	9.7

Chart 1

Deaths due to heart disease with reference to the consumption of saturated fats (Seven Country Study)

Coronary deaths

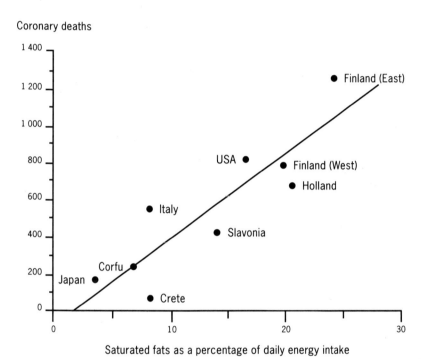

Saturated fats as a percentage of daily energy intake

(Sources: OMS – OECD)

Chart 2

Deaths due to heart disease with reference to the consumption of milk products (men and women)

Coronary deaths (1988)

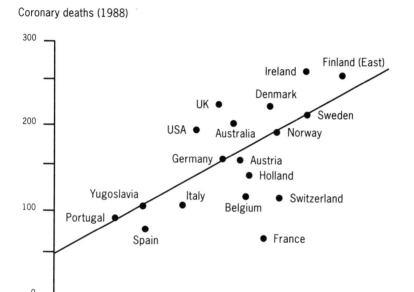

Calorific value of milk products

(Sources: OMS – OECD)

225

Chart 3

Deaths due to heart disease with reference to the consumption of cheese (men and women)

Coronary deaths (1988)

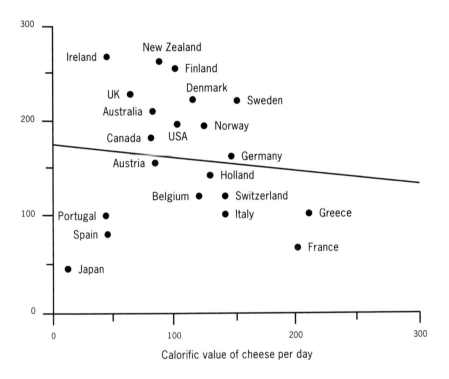

Calorific value of cheese per day

(Sources: OMS – OECD)

Chart 4

Deaths due to heart disease with reference to the consumption of vegetables, fruit and vegetable fats by men

Coronary deaths (1989)

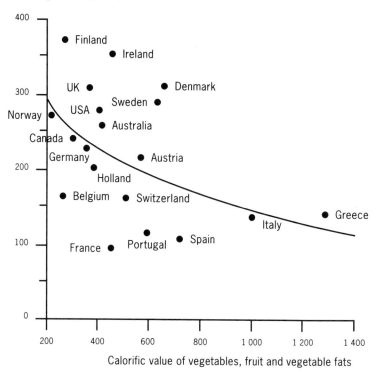

Calorific value of vegetables, fruit and vegetable fats

(Sources: OMS – OECD)

Chart 5

Deaths due to heart disease with reference to the consumption of alcohol by men

Coronary deaths (1989)

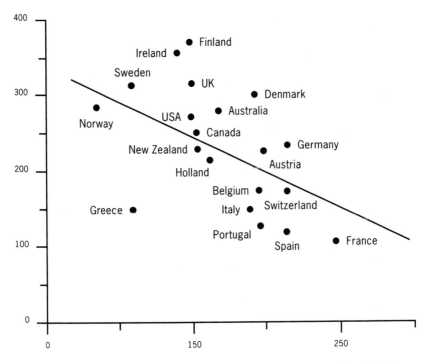

Daily consumption of alcohol in calories (1 gram alcohol = 7 calories)

(*Source: OMS*)

Chart 6

Deaths due to heart disease with reference to the consumption of wine by men

Coronary deaths (1989)

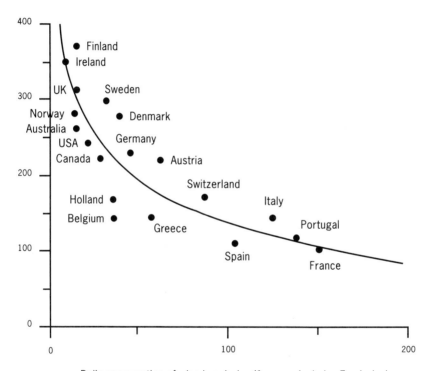

Daily consumption of wine in calories (1 gram alcohol = 7 calories)

(Source: OMS)

Chart 7

**Relationship between the consumption of alcohol and death
of 276,000 Americans from different causes**

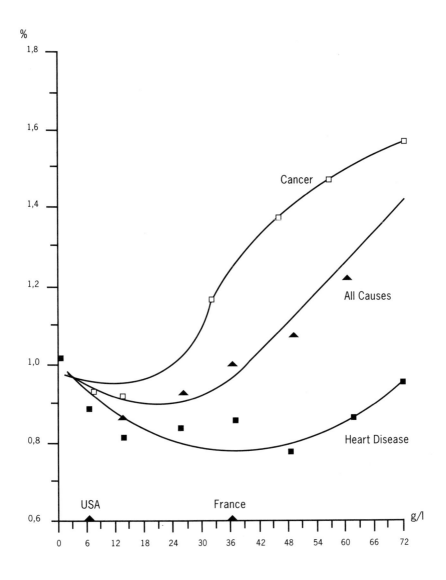

Adapted from Bofetta and Garfinkel, 1990

Chart 8

Relative risk of death associated with the consumption of alcohol

Relative risk

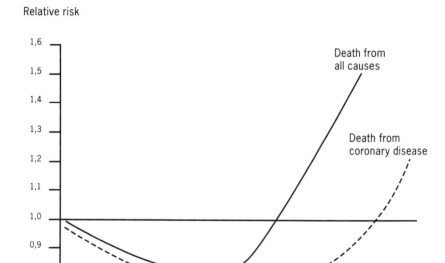

Glasses of alcohol consumed per day

(Source: H. Schlienger)

231

BIBLIOGRAPHY

Abadie JB *Le vin en théapeutique de l'Antiquité à nos jours*

Aigrain P *La consommation de vin en France en 1990* Montpellier, ONVINS-INRA, 1991

Albert JP *Le vin dans les texte sacrés,* Paris Bull de l'OIV,1987

Angelico F *Habitual alcohol consumption and HDL cholesterol* Ann Nutr Metab, 1982, 26, 73-76, 45

Archambault JC *Alcoologie,* Paris, Masson, 1995

Aron JP *Le mageur du XIXe siècle,* Paris, Laffont, 1973

Arpentine GN *Effets physiologiques du vin: intérêt dans le domaine de la santé,* Bull de l'OIV,juin 1994

Balmes JL *Evolution des comportements des adolescents vi-à-vis des boissons alcoolisées en France,* Revue de œnologues, no.71

Barrucand D *Alcoologie,* Lab. Riom, 1988

Baspeyras M *Le vin médecin,* Miverve, 1986

Bauza T *Les amines biogènes du vin, métabolisme, toxicité,* Bull de l'OIV, 1995, 767-768, 42-67

Belda E *Alcoolisme: épidémiologie, pathologie, dépistage,* Cah Nutr Diet, 1995, 30, 3 195-200

Berteilli AAE *Antiplatelet activity of synthetic and natural resveratrol in red wines,* Int J Tissue, 1995, XVII, 1-3

Bertin J *Le vin et la santé: promouvoir l'éducation et la qualité,* Journée viticole, 1990, 18, 107, 1-4

Bihaut S *Le vin authentique,* Paris, Sang de la terre, 1993

Blanchet J *Les courtiers-jurés picqueurs de vins dans l'histoire de Paris,* Paris, Daniel Lestrade, 1985

Bologne JC *Histoire morale et culturelle de nos boissons,* Paris, Laffont, 1991

Bonal F *Le livre d'or du champagne,* Lausanne, Ed. Du Grand Pont, 1984

235

Bonal F   *Les vertus thérapeutiques du champagne,* Paris, Artulen 1990

Bouix JC   *Le sevrage alcoolique ambulatoire en médecine générale,* Rev du Prat, 1996, 10, 325, 11-15

Boulet D   *L'évolution des comportements de consommation du vin en France,* Revue des œnologues, no.77

Bourzeix M   *La place du vin dans l'hygiène alimentaire,* in *De l'alcoolisme au bien-boire* by G. Caro, Paris, L'Harmattan, 1990

Bourzeix M   *Influence des polyphénols du raisin et du vine sur la santé,* Actualités diet., 1993, 371-376

Bradbury J   *Grapes are good for you, but leave the skins,* Lancet, 1997, 349, 107

Braitberg JM   *Le scandale des vins frelatés,* Monaco, Ed. Du Rocher, 1993

Braquet P   *Protective effect of flavonoids against the non enzymatic degradation of collagen by oxy-free-radicals,* CR Groupe Polyphénols, 1982, 11, 496-507

Bravo L   *Degradation of polyphenols in intestinal tract. Effect on colonic fermentation and fecal output,* Br J Nutr 1994, 71, 6, 933-946

Brun S   *Les propriétés biologiques des constituants non alcooliques du vin,* Cah Nutr Diet, 1995, 30, 4, 224-229

Camargo CA   *Type A behaviour pattern and alcohol intake in middle-aged men,* Psychosmot Med 48, 1986, 575-581

Carles J   *La chimie du vin,* Paris, PUF, Que-sais-je? no.908, 1877

Caro G   *De l'alcoolisme au bien-boire,* Paris, L'Harmatta, 1990

Casswell S   *Does alcohol advertising have an impact on the public health?* Drug and Alcohol Rev., 1995, 14, 395-404

Castro JM   *Moderate alcohol intake and spontaneous eating patterns of humans: evidence of unregulated supplementation,* Am J Clin Nutr, 1990, 52, 246-253

Christanse C — *Wine for type 2 diabetic patients?* Diabet Med, 1993, 10, 10, 958-961

Clifford AJ — *Delayed tumour onset in transgenic mice fed an amino acid-based diet supplemented with red wine solids,* Am J Clin Nutr, 1996, 64, 748-756

Constant R — *Le vin et la longévité,* Bordeaux, Thèse 1935

Contaldo F — *Short-term effects of moderate alcohol consumption on lipid metabolism and energy balance in normal men,* Metabolism, 1989, 38, 2, 166-171

Cook JD — *The effect of red and white wines on nonhemeion absorption in humans,* Am J clin Nutr, 1995, 61, 800-804

Cornemere C — *Les vins de France,* Paris, Nathan, 1995

Costa Magna M — *Les femmes et l'alcool,* Paris, Denoël, 1981

Criqui MH — *Does diet or alcohol explain the French paradox?,* Lancet, 1994, 344, 1719-1723

Cuny M — *Historique de la consommation d'alcool des Français,* Paris, Thèse de Médecine, 1980

Dally S — *La dépandance à l'alcool éthelique, Problème psychologique ou phénomène biologique?,* Concours Med., 1991, 113, 6, 4555-458

Da Silva R — *Oxygen-free radical scavenger capacity in aqueous models of different procyanidisn from grape seeds,* J Agric Food Chem, 1991, 39, 1549

David JP — *Vin, santé, plaisir de vivre: utopie ou défi?,* Revue des œnologues, 1992, XXIX, 70, 47-50

David JP — *Vin et alimentation: la place du vin dan l'hygiène alimentaire,* Paris, Bull. OIV, 1992, 739-740, 727-743

David JP — *L'amour et la loi,* Mâcon, talk 1993

Day A — *Cardioprotective effect of red wine may be mediated by urate,* Clin Chem, 1995, 41, 9, 1319-1320

Demrow HS — *Administration of wine and grape juice inhibits in vivo* *platelet activity and thrombosis in stenosed canine coronary arteries,* Circulation, 1995, 91, 1182-1188

Deynoux J *Thérapeutique du vin,* Bordeaux, Thèse de Médecine, 1987

D'Houtaud A *Alcohol consumption in France: production, consumption, morbidity and mortality, prevention and education in the last three decades,* Advances in alcohol and substance abuse, 8, 1889, 19-44

Dion R *Histoire de la vigne et du vin en France des origines au XIXe siècle,* Paris, Flammarion, 1977

Doll R *Mortality in relation to consumption of alcohol: 13 years observations on mle Dritish doctors,* BMJ, 309, 1994, 911-918

Domenach G *Eloge de l'ivresse,* Paris, Albin Michel, 1981

Dougnac *Le vin,* Thèse de Médecine, Bordeaux, 1933

Ducimetiere P *Coronary heart disease in middle-aged Frenchmen. Comparisons between Paris Prospective Study, Seven Countries and Pooling Project",* Lancet, 1, 1990, 1346-1350

Ducimetiere P *Le paradoxe français,mythe ou réalité,* Cah Nutr Diet, 1995, 30, 2, 78-81

Dugoua B *La vigne, le vine e les buveurs à Rome dans l'Antiquité,* Bordeaux, Thèse de Médecine, 1980

Dumas J *Activité levuricide du leucocyanidol en présence de cuivre,* Ann Inst Pasteur, 1971, 121, 69-73

Dumay R *La mort du vin,* Paris, Stock, 1976

Duncan BB *Association of the waist-to-hip ration is different with wine than beer or hard liquor concumption,* Am J Epidemiol, 1995, 142, 1034-1038

Durand Y *L'imaginaire de l'alcoolisme,* Paris, Ed. Universitaires, 1972

Durbec R *L'esprit du vin. Santé et thérapie par le vin biologique,* Gran-Lancy, Jouvence, 1993

Enjalbert H   *Histoire de la vigne et du vin. L'avènement de la qualité,* Paris, Borda, 1975

Eylaud JM   *Vin et santé,* Paris, Ed. La Nouvelle diffusion du liver, 1960

Farchi G   *Alcohol and mortality in the Italian rural cohorts of Seven Countries Study,* Int J Epidemiol, 21, 1992, 74-82

Fitzpatrick DF   *La peau du raisin aurait un effet bénéfique sur le maladies cardio-vasculaires,* Journée viticole, 1994, 18, 816, 8

Formica JV   *Biology of quercitin and related bioflavenoids,* Food Chem. Toxic., 1995, 33, 1061-1080

Fouquet P   *Le roman de l'alcool,* Paris, Seghers, 1986

Fouquet P   *Histoire de l'alcool,* Paris, PUF, Que sais-je? no.2521, 1990

François A   *Les aspects nutritionnels du savoir-boire,* Bull de l'OIV, 1991, 64, 725-726,545

François A   *Le glycérol dan l'alimentation,* Acad d'agric de France, 1994, 80, 2, 63-76

Frankel EN   *Inhibition of oxidation of human low-density lipoproteins by phenolic substances in red wine,* Lancet, 341, 1993, 454-457

Frankel EN   *Principal phenolic phytochemicals in selected California wines and their antioxidant activity in inhibiting oxidation of human low-density lipoproteins,* J Agric Food Chem, 1995, 43, 890-894

Frezza M   *High blood alcohol levels in women,* New Engl j Med, 1989, 322, 95-99

Fuhrman B   *Consumption of red wine with meals reduces the susceptibility of human plasma and low density lipoproteins to lipid peroxidation,* Am J Clin Nutr, 1995, 61, 549-554

Gaignard J-Y   *L'alcoologie en pratique quotidienne,* Lab MERAM, 1992

Garrier G   *Le vin des historiens,* Suze la Rousse, Université du vin, 1990

239

Garrier G *Histoire sociale et culturelle du vin,*Paris, Bordas, 1995

Gautier J-F *Le vin à travers les âges, de la mythologie à l'œnologie,* Bordeaux, LCF, 1989

Gautier J-F *Histoire du vin,* Paris, PUF, Que sais-je? no.2676, 1992

Gautier J-F *Le vin et ses fraudes,* Paris, PUF, Que sais-je? no.3001, 1995

Gaziano JM *Moderate alcohol intake, increased levels of high density lipoproteins and its subfraction and decreased risk of myocardial infarction,*N Engl J Med, 1993, 329, 1829-1834

Genevoix L *Propriétés physiologiques du vin,* Cah Nutr ed Diet 1982, 2, 87-89

Georgescu PL *Effets inhibiteurs des extraits de vin sur la formation des produits glycatés de la réaction de Maillard,* Med et Nutr 1996, 32, 3, 117-119

Ghalim N *Influence de l'alchool sur les lipides plasmatiques et l'arthérogémèse,* Presse Med, 1991, 20, 11, 507-512

Gin H *Short-term effect of red wine on insulin requirement and glucose tolerance in diabetic patients,* Diabetes Care, 1992, 15, 4, 546-548

Gin H *La consommation modérée de vin a-t-elle une influence sur l'equilibre glycémique du patient diabétique?,* Rev Nutr Prat, 1993, 7, 21

Girre L *Le pouvoir antiherpétique in vitro des feuilles de vigne rouge,* Filoterapia, 1990, LXI, 3, 201-205

Glories J-F *Les polyphénols du raisin et du vin,* Rev Nutr Prat, Dietecom 93, 1993, 7, 21-25

Goldberg DM *Does wine work?* Clin Chem, 1995, 41, 1, 14-16

Goldberg DM *More on antioxidant activity of resveratrol in red wine,* Clin Chem, 1996, 42, 1, 113-114

Gronbaek M *Mortality associated with moderate intakes of wine, beer or spirits,* BMJ, 310, 1995, 1165-69

Hagiage M   *Alcool, HDL et maladie coronarienne,* Cah Nutr Diet, 990, XXV, 6, 402-408

Halpern GM   *The effect of white wine upon pulmonary function of asthmatic subjects,* Ann Allergy, 1985, 55, 5, 686-690

Hein H   *Alcohol consumption, serum low density protein cholesterol concentration, and risk of ischaemic heart disease: 6 years follow up in the Copenhagen male study,* BMJ, 1996, 312, 736-741

Hendriks H   *Effect of moderated dose of alcohol with evening meal on fibrionic factors,* BMJ, 1994, 308

Hennekens CH   *Effects of beer, wine and liquor in coronary deaths,* JAMA, 1979, 242, 18 1973-1974

Hertog MGL   *Dietary antioxydant flavonoids and risk of coronary heart disease: the Zutphen Elderly Study,* Lancet, 1993, 342, 1007-1011

Hertog MGL   *Flavonoid intake and long-term risk of coronary heart disease and cancer in the Seven Countires Study,* Arch Inter Med, 1995, 155, 381-386

Hillbom ME   *What supports the role of alcohol as a risk factor for stroke?,* Acta Med Scand, 717, 1987, suppl, 93-106

Hillemand B   *Composante génétique de l'alcoolisme,* Med et Nutr, 1991, XXVII, 6, 348-352

Holbrook T   *A prospective study of alcohol consumption and bone mineral density,* BMJ, 1993, 306

Holloway FA   *Low-dose alcohol effects on human behaviour and performance,* Alcohol, drugs and driving, 1995, 11, 1, 39-56

Huas D   *Prévalence du risque et des maladies liés à l'alcool dans la clientèle adulte du généraliste,* Rev du Prat, 1993, 7, 203, 39-44

Hurt RD   *Plasma lipids and apolipoprotein A! and A' levels in alcoholic patients,* Am J Clin Nutr, 1986, 43, 521-529

Izou L   *La défense du vin,* Paris, 1906

Jackson R   *Does recent alcohol consumption reduce the risk of acute myocardial infarction and coronary death in regular drinkers?*, Am J of Epidemiol, 1992, 136, 7, 819-824

Jackson R   *The relationship between alcohol and coronary heart disease: is there a protective effect?*, Curr Opin Lipidol, 1993, 4, 21-26

Jaham MR   *Vin, mon ami,* Paris, Laffont, 1991

Jalkunen RJK   *First-pass metabolism of ethanol,* Life Sci, 1985, 37, 567-573

Johnson H   *Histoire mondiale du vin,* Paris, Hachette, 1991

Jones Fr   *Bon, vin, bon cœur, bonne santé,* Ed de l'Homme, Montréal, 1995

Keys A   *How to eat and stay well, the Mediterranean way,* New York, Doubleday, 1975

Keys A   *Wine, garlic and coronary heart disease in seven countries,* Lancet, 1980, 141-154

Keys A   *The Seven Countries study: 2289 deaths in 15 years,* Prev Med, 13, 1984, 141-154

Kinsella JE   *Possible mechanisms for the protective role of antioxidants in wine and plant foods,* Food Technology, 1993-3, 85-89

Klag M   *Alcohol and cardio-vascular disease,* Annual report of WELCH, John Hopkins University

Klatsky AL   *The relationship between alcoholic beverage use and other traits to blood pressure,* Circulation, 1986, 73, 628-636

Klatsky AL   *Alcohol and mortality,* Ann Intern Med, 117, 1992, 646-654

Knekt P   *Flavonoid intake and coronary mortality in Finland: a cohort study,* BMJ, 1996, 312, 478-481

Kondo K   *Inhibitions of oxidation of low-density lipoprotein with red wine,* Lancet, 344, 1994, 1152

Konowalchuk J   *Virus inactivation by grapes and wines,* Appl Environ Microbiol, 1976, 32, 6, 757-763

Lachiver M   *Vins, vignes et vignerons. Histoire du vignoble français,* Paris, Fayard, 1988

Lang T   *Mieux prendre en compte l'obésité et l'alcoolisme,* Tempo Medical, 1992, 453, 9-10

Langer RD   *Lipoproteins and blood pressure as biologic pathways for the effect of moderate alcohol consumption on coronary heart disease,* Circulation, 85, 1992, 910-915

Laparra J   *Etude pharmacocinétique des oligomères procyanidoliques totaux du raisin,* Acta Ther, 1978, 4, 233-246

Laparra J   *Vin et santé,* Rev Fr d'Œnologie, 1993, 143, 55-57

Laparra J   *Etude des oligomères procyanoliques sur le cobaye carancé en vitamine C,* Bull Soc Parm, 118, 7-13, 60

Lazarus NB   *Change in alcohol consumption and risk of death from all causes and from ischaemic heart disease,* BMJ, 1991, 303, 553-556

Lea AGH   *The procyanidins of white grapes and wines,* Am J Enol Vitic, 1979, 30, 4, 289-300

Le Bail V   *Diététique et alcoolisme: habitudes, risques, conseils,* Cah Nutr Diet, 1991 XXVI, 6, 432-434

Lejoyeux M   *Bases biologiques de l'appétence à l'alcool,* Synapse, 1994, 104, 4-6

Lenz HJ   *Wine and five percent ethanol are potent stimulants of gastric acid secretion in humans,* Gastroenterology, 1983, 85, 1082-1087

Lipton RI   *The effect of moderate alcohol use on the relationship between stress and depression,* Am J Public Health, 1994, 84, 12, 1913-1917

Mahe N   *Le mythe de Bacchus,* Paris, Fayard, 1992

Manson J   *The primary prevention of myocardial infarction,* The New Engl J of Med, 1992, 326, 21

Marechal C   *L'alcool et les jeunes,* Paris, Programme 7, 1981

Marmot M   *Alcohol and cardiovascular disease. The status of the U shaped curve,* BMJ, 1991, 303, 565-568

Masquelier J   *Interactions boissons alcoolisées-medicaments,* Ann Hyg L Fr Med et Nutr, 1975, 11, 4, 283-289

Masquelier J   *Effets physiologiques des constituants non alcoooliques du vin,* Cah Nutr et Diet, 1976, 5, 4, 68

Masquelier J   *Le vin et la santé,* Paris, Bull de l'OIV, 1976, 586, 1023-1035

Masquelier J   *Action bactéricide et antivirale du vin – 10e Congrès des Sociétés savantes,* Bordeaux, 1979, fasc, II, 447-457

Masquelier J   *Pycnogénols,* Bull Soc Parm, Bordeaux, 1979, 118, 95-108

Masquelier J   *Stabilisation du collagène par les oligomères procyanidolique,* Acta Ther, 1981, 7, 101-105

Masquelier J   *Fungicide properties of certain components of the grape and wine,* Symposium "Wine, health and society", 13-14 nov.1981, San Francisco

Masquelier J   *Les Procyanidols du vin,* Bull de l'OIV, 1991, 88-93

Masquelier J   *La vigne, plante médicinale – Naissance d'une thérapeutique,* Paris, Bull de l'OIV, 1992, 65, 733-734, 175-196

Matthews T   *Wine: prescription for good health,* Wine spectator, 1994, 18, 20, 36-48

Maxwell S   *Red wine and antioxydant activity in serum,* Lancet, 344, 1994, 193-194

Maury E   *Notre vin quotidien,* Paris, Ed. Universitaires, 1987

Maury E   *La Médecine par le vin,* Paris, Artulen, 1988

Menon LG   *Inhibition of lung metastasis in mice induced by B 16F10 melanoma cells by polyphenolic compounds,* Cancer Letters, 1995, 95, 221-225

Mesnier J   *Le vin et la santé,* Journée viticole, 1991, 18, 319, 1-6

Messing B   *Alcool et métabolisme énergétique,* Cah Nutr diet, 1995, 30, 4, 211-215

244

Miller GJ   *Alcohol consumption: protection against coronary heart disease and risk to health,* Inter J of Epidemiology, 1990, 19, 4, 923-930

Mirouze J   *Vin et santé,* Rev Fr Œnol, 1985, 97, 5-12

Mizuno T   *Inhibitory effect of tannic acid sulphate and related sulphates on infectivity, cytopathic effect, and giant cell formation of human immunodeficiency virus,* Planta Med, 1992, 58, 6, 535-539

Moore JG   *Effect of wine on gastric emptying in humans,* Gastroenterology, 1981, 6, 1072-1075

Morisot D   *Evaluation d'une action éducative sur le risque d'alcool no.2,* Cahiers de l'IREB, 1995, 2, 175-179

Naoum-Grappe V   *La culture de l'ivresse, Essai de phénoménologiee historique,* Paris, Quai Voltaire, 1991

Nakashima H   *Inhibition of human immunodeficiency vital replication by tannins and related compounds,* Antiviral Res, 1992, 18, 1, 91-103

Napo F   *La révolte des vignerons,* Toulouse, Private, 1971

Nourisson D   *Le buveur du XIXe siècle,* Paris, Albin Michel, 1990

Okuda T   *Chemistry and biological activity of tannins in medicinal plants,* Economic and medicinal research, 1991, 5, 129-165

Ole HH   *Alcohol consumption, serum low density lipoprotein cholesterol concentration, and risk of ischaemic heart disease: six year follow-up in the Copenhagen male study,* BMJ, 1996, 312, 736-741

Paille F   *Sucre ou alcool, faut-il choisir?* Informations diététiques, 93, 2, 1-5

Pasteur L   *Etudes sur le vin,* Paris, 1866

Pelicier Y   *Les ivresses,* Bordeaux, L'Esprit du temps, 1993

Perdue L   *Le paradoxe français,* Avignon, A. Barthelemy, 1995

245

Petersen WL   *Effect of intragastric infusions of ethanol and wine on serum gastrin contration and gastric acid secretion,* Gastroenterology, 1986, 91, 1390-1395

Peynaud E   *Le goût du vin,* Dunod, 1980

Paynaud E   *Le vin et les jours,* Paris, Dunod, 1988

Portmann G   *Les vins de Bordeaux sont vins de santé,* Bull As Med pour l'étude scientifique du vin et du raisin, 1956, 1

Pradignac A   *caractéristiques nutritionnelles d'un échantillon de personnes âgéesvivant à domicile dans le département du Bas-Rhin,* Enquête Alsanut 3e age, Cah Nutr Diet, 1993, 28, 236-244

Puissais J   *Le vin se met à table,* Paris, Marcel Valtat, 1981

Regan TJ   *Alcohol and the cardiovascular system,* JAMA, 1990, 264, 377-381

Renault-Roger C   *Vitamine P, bioflavanoides ou facteur C": réévaluation d'un concept,* Cah Nutr Diet, 1986, 231, 5, 359-360

Remesy C   *Intérêt ntritionnel del flavonoides,* Med et Nutr, 1996, 32, 1, 17-37

Renaud S   *Influence of long-term diet modification on platelet function and composition in Moselle farmers,* Am J Clin Nutr, 43, 1986, 136-150

Renaud S   *Wine, alcohol, platelets and the French Paradox for coronary heart disease,* Lancet, 339, 1992, 1523-1526

Renaud S   *Alcohol and platelet aggregation: The Caerphilly prospective heart disease study,* Am J Clin Nutr, 55, 1992, 1012-1017

Renaud S   *Alcohol drinking and coronary heart disease,* Health Issues related to Alcohol Consumption, PM Verschuren, Ed ILSI Press, Washington, 1993, p.81-123

Renaud S   *The French Paradox: vegetables or wine,* Circulation, 90, 1994, 3118

Renaud S   *The Cretan Mediterranean diet for prevention of coronary heart disease,* Am J Clin Nutr 61 (suppl), 1995, 1360S-1367S

Renaud S   *Le régime santé,* Paris, Odile Jacob, 1995

Renaud S   *Effects of alcohol on platelet functions,* Clinica Chim
Acta, 1996, 246, 77-89

Renvoise G   *Le monde du vin: art ou bluff,* Rodez, Ed. Du Rouergue,
1994

Ricci G   *Alcohol intake and coronary risk factors in a population
group of Rome,* Nutr Metab, 1977, 21, suppl.1, 157-159

Ridker PM   *Association of moderate alcohol consumption and
plasma concentration of endogenous tissue-type
plasminogen activator,* JAMA, 1994, 272, 929-933

Rijkey B   *Red wine consumption and oxidation of low density
proteins,* Lancet, 1995, 345, April, 325-326

Rimm EB   *Alcohol and mortality,* Lancet, 338, 1991, 1073-1074

Rimm EB   *Review of moderate alcohol consumption and reduced
risk of coronary heart disease: is the effect due to beer,
wine, or spirits?,* BMJ, 1996, 312, 731-736

Romani A   *Les composants polyphénoliques de caractère flavonoide
des raisins et du vin,* Bull de l'OIV, June 1994

Rueff B   *Alcoologie clinique,* Paris, Flammarion Médecine, 1989

Ruf J-C   *Platelet rebound effect of alcohol withdrawal and wine
drinking in rats. Relation to tannins and lipid peroxidation,*
Arterioscl Throm Vasc Biol, 15, 1995, 140-144

Saint-Leger AS   *Factors associated with cardiac mortality in developed
countries with particular reference to consumption of
wine,* Lancet, 1979, 1017-1020

Sasaki S   *Wine and non wine alcohol: differential effect on all
cause and cause specific mortality,* Nutr Metab
Cardiovasc Dis, 1994, 4, 177-182

Schlienger JL   *Consumption d'alcohol et statut nutritionnel,* Rev de
Gériatrie, March 1992

Schlienger JL   *Consommation modéré d'alcool et maladies cardio-
vasculaires,* Diet et Med, 1994, 4, 153-159

Schlienger JL   *La consommation de vin a-t-elle des effets bénéfiques?* Rev de Nutr Prat, 1994, 8, 25-28

Schlienger JL   *Effets de la consommation alimentaire et d'alcool sur les paramètres lipidiques d'une population âgée vivant a domicile,* Cah Nutr Diet, 1996, 31, 138-143

Seigneur M   *Effect of consumption of alcohol, white wine and red wine on platelet function and serum lipids,* J of Applied Cardiology, 1990, 5

Servard D   *Les moines et le vin,* Pygmalion-Gérard Watelet, 1982

Sharpe PC   *Effect of red wine consumption on lipoprotein (a) and other risk factors for atherosclerosis,* Q J Med, 1995, 88, 101-108

Simonetti P   *Evaluation of the effect of alcohol consumption on erythrocyte lipids and vitamins in a healthy population,* Alcohol Clin Exp Res, 1995, 19, 2, 517-522

Singer MV   *Low concentrations of ethanol stimulate gastric acid secretion independent of gastrin release in humans,* Gastroenterology, 1984, 86, 1254-1261

Skog OJ   *Public health consequences of the J-curve hypothesis of alcohol problems,* Addiction, 1996, 91, 3, 325-337

Sournia J-C   *Histoire de l'alcoolisme,* Paris, Flammarion, 1986

Stampfer M-J   *A prospective study of moderate alcohol drinking and risk of diabetes in women,* Am J Epidemiol, 1988, 128, 3, 549-558

Stroewsand GS   *Inhibition by wine of tunorigenesis induced by ethylcarbamate in mice,* Food Chem toxicol, 1991, 29, 5, 291-295

Suhonen O   *Alcohol consumption and sudden coronary death in middle-aged Finnish men,* Acta Med Scand, 221, 1987, 335-341

Sulzky SI   *Descriptors of alcohol consumption among non institutionalized non alcoholic elderly,* J Am Nutr, 1990, 9, 326-331

Takeshi M   *Structure and antiherpetic activity among tannins,* Phytochemistry, 24, 2245

Taskinen MR   *Alcohol-induced changes in serum lipoproteins and in their metabolism,* Am Heart J, 1987, 113, 458-466

Teissedre PL   *Inhibition of in-vitro human LDL oxidation by phenolic substances from grapes and wines,* J Sci Food Agric, 1996, 70, 55-61

Torel J   *Antioxidant activity of flanonoids and reactivity with peroxy radical,* Phytochemistry, 1986, 25, 383

Toussaint-Samat M *Histoire naturelle et morale de la nourriture,* Paris, Bordas, 1987

Tran Ky   *Les vertus thérapeutiques du Bordeaux,* Paris, Artulen, 1991

Tran Ky   *Les vertus médicinales du Bourgogne,* Besançon, Cètre, 1995

Tremolieres J   *Physiochimie et biochimie de l'oxydation de l'alcool dans l'organisme. Du don usage du vin,* Paris, PUF, 1973

Troup GJ   *Free radicals in red wine, but not in white?,* Free-Radic Res, 1994, 20, 1, 63-68

Turner T   *Beer and wine of geriatric patients,* JAMA, 1973, 12, 222, 7, 46

Verschuren M   *Serum total cholesterol and long-term coronary heart disease mortality in different cultures,* JAMA, 1995, 274, 131-136

Vinson JA   *Phenol antioxidant index: comparative antioxidant effectiveness of red and white wines,* J Agric Food Chem, 1995, 43, 401-403

Waterhouse A   *Inhibition of human LDL oxidation by resveratrol,* Lancet, 1993, 341

Weill J   *Pour une lecture critique de la loi de Lederman,* IREB, 1993

Weill J   *Factors predictive of alcohol consumption in a representative sample of French male teenagers: a five-year prospective study,* Drug and Alcohol Dep, 1994, 35, 45-50

Weisse ME   *Wine as a digestive aid, comparative antimicrobial effects of bismuth salicylate and red and white wine,* BMJ, 1995, 311, 1657-1660

Whitehead TP   *Effect of red wine ingestion on the antioxidant capacity of serum,* Clin Chem, 995, 41, 1, 32-35

Yano K   *Coffee, alcohol and risk of coronary heart disease among Japanese men living in Hawaii,* New Engl J Med, 297, 1977, 405-409

Ziegler O   *Consommation d'alcool et lipoprotéines plasmatiques,* Cah Nutr Diet, 1995, 30, 4, 216-223

American Council on Science and Health, *The responsible use of alcohol. Defining the parameters of moderation,* New York, A.C.S.H., 1991

Attitudes et comportements des jeunes Français face à l'alcool, Doc IREB, 1991

De la composition du raisin et du vin et des effets de leur consommation, Paris, Bull de l'OIV, 1989

Le vin dans les textes sacrés et les cultures méditerranéennes, Paris, Bull de l'OIV, 1988

La vigne et le vin, L'ARC, Cahiers méditerranéens, Paris, Ed. Duponchelle, 1990

Sécurité routière: les chiffres clés en 1995, Documents du ministère des Transports, 15.03.96

Synthèses et conclusions du groupe intergouvernemental de la F.A.O. sur la consommation de vin et la santé, Paris, Bull de l'OIV, 1994

Vigne, raisin, vin et santé, Paris, Bull de l'OIV, 1993

Le vin, plaisir et santé, Entretiens de Belley, 1993

Vin et civilisation, Colloque du CILOP, Paris-Turin, 1984

Vignes et vins, Historia, no.468, December 1985

Vin et santé, Talk on the 14.05.93 at Aix-en-Provence

Vin et santé, L'Impatient, 1993, hors-série no.5